# THE
# EXPECTANT
# FATHER

**Cartoons by Mel Calman**

# THE
# EXPECTANT
# FATHER

by

**Betty Parsons**

## A PRACTICAL GUIDE
## TO SHARING PREGNANCY
## AND CHILDBIRTH

## PAPERFRONTS

**ELLIOT RIGHT WAY BOOKS,
KINGSWOOD, SURREY, U.K.**

Made and Printed in Great Britain by
Cox and Wyman Ltd, Reading.

# FOREWORD

Betty Parsons has helped many hundreds of husbands and wives to understand pregnancy and labour. She has allayed the phobias, irrational worries and mysteries that have grown up round this natural event. Her book fulfils a long-felt need – it explains simply but intelligently how a husband can support his wife during this important and happy period of their lives, which all too often can be spoilt by misunderstanding and superstition.

Support from the medical profession, an intimate knowledge of her subject and many years of teaching young parents are only contributory to her amazing success and achievements, which owe most to a remarkable personality capable of instilling confidence in all who come to her classes.

With the publication of her book for expectant fathers she reaches out to all those who have not benefited from her teaching at first hand.

JOHN BOSTOCK
M.R.C.O.G.

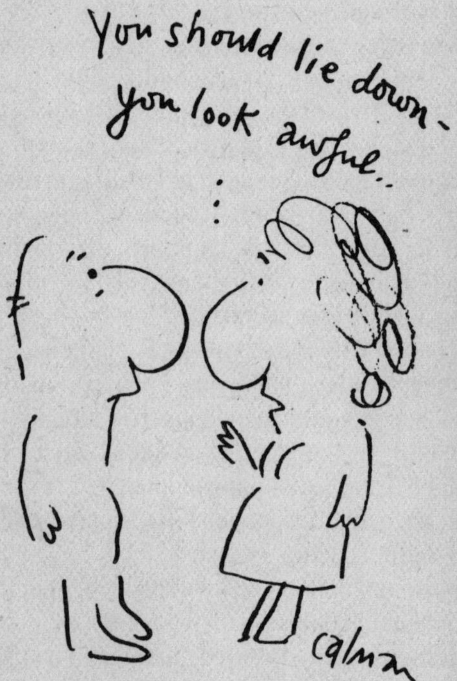
You should lie down-
you look awful...
calman

# ACKNOWLEDGEMENTS

I have received much help from a number of people in the preparation of this book. I am grateful to them all. I would like especially to thank Mr. John Bostock, M.R.C.O.G. for his helpful suggestions and for writing a foreword, Mr. Peter Ford for bringing his interest and expertise to the editing of the book, Mr. Leo Cavendish who first suggested it be written; and C. Howard and Partners and Robert Yeatman Ltd. who were responsible for the original edition.

I would also like to acknowledge my debt to the late Drs. Grantly Dick Read and Fernand Lamaze, on whose work much of my teaching is based.

# CONTENTS

# ILLUSTRATIONS

# INTRODUCTION

For both man and woman pregnancy can be a very difficult period. It has its joyous moments of anticipation and preparation, but it has too its moments of depression and difficulties. It can put a great strain on a relationship, and depending on the way one adjusts to it, a relationship can be weakened or strengthened and matured.

Over the years I have taught several thousand women about pregnancy and childbirth. During my course of classes I give a Fathers' Evening to which both expectant fathers and mothers come. So many times girls have said to me afterwards: 'I can't tell you what a difference it has made to my husband now that he understands what it is all about. Since the Fathers' Evening my husband feels so much more involved. He feels it is *his* baby as well.' 'You should give the Fathers' Evening much earlier on... If only he had understood all this from the beginning.'

With this latter remark I entirely agree. But I wonder how many men would agree to go to a Fathers' Evening during early pregnancy. I suspect very few. It is only the interest evoked by their wives relating what happens in classes and the close proximity of the birth that makes them (sometimes very reluctantly) agree to spend an evening learning about the whole process of childbirth.

That is why this book has been written – in the hope that men will read it early during their wives' pregnancy, and by understanding more about it they will be able to help not only their wives, but also themselves to adjust to one of the greatest changes that will occur in their lives.

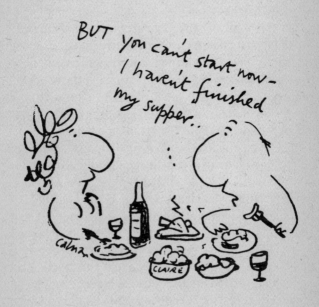

BUT you can't start now – I haven't finished my supper..

# PART I

# THE ANTE-NATAL PERIOD

# 1

# Blame it on the Hormones

Your wife is pregnant. If it is for the first time a new era in your life is starting. Many different emotions crowd in: pleasure, fear, excitement, apprehension and probably the first inklings of the responsibility that parenthood will bring. It takes time for the reality of the situation to sink in for both the mother and the father-to-be. The birth of their baby is something that will not happen until nine months after conception, and in the early days of pregnancy it seems to have little reality. On the surface everything goes on much as usual but underneath are the stirrings of great changes that will inevitably affect their lives.

Immediately a woman becomes pregnant, hormonal changes start to occur in her body. Hormones are the secretions of the endocrine glands, and to a great extent they govern what we are – our size, shape and temperament. The activities of the hormones can make us happy or sad, energetic or slow-moving. From conception and during pregnancy hormones play a very special role both physically and emotionally. Much depends on their correct balance and function, and their activity is beyond our conscious control.

This last fact needs to be stressed, for your wife

may often feel guilty because she cannot control the fluctuations of mood that she finds herself experiencing during pregnancy. One day she is bright, happy and excited, full of optimistic anticipation at the prospect of having her baby. The next she may be depressed and crying, wishing she had never got pregnant at all. But guilt is a very negative emotion, and it always builds tensions in the person who experiences it and so only aggravates the situation.

## A SENSE OF HUMOUR

For this reason pregnancy is a time that demands a sense of humour. A woman needs to accept herself as she is and to be able to smile at the extraordinary things she sometimes finds herself doing. And how much easier it is for her to bring this light-hearted attitude to the situation when there is someone with whom to share her laughter.

It is well known that when we feel depressed or angry we tend to vent our bad mood on those who are nearest and dearest to us. Never is this more true than during pregnancy, and it is not easy for a man to accept his pregnant wife's strange behaviour and emotional outbursts unless he understands what produces them. The cause may seem so trivial and illogical.

What one day would make her laugh, the next day will be the cause of uncontrollable tears. Remarks meant to be kind and helpful are taken as criticisms, and things may reach the point when

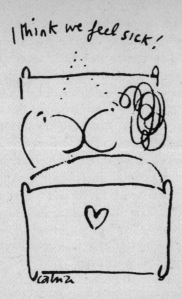

you wonder what has become of the sweet-natured girl you married! It is all very difficult to accept, unless you understand the effects that hormonal change can have on a woman's emotions during pregnancy. In pregnancy a woman becomes what I would call 'emotionally fragile', especially during the first and last three months of pregnancy. So many women say to me: 'I feel my character has changed. Will I ever be the same again?' Of course they will, as we shall see.

There was one girl who rang me up to plead: 'Please speak to him and tell him I don't mean it.' She was going through an extreme bout of irritability and, of course, the person who was the target for her ill humour was her unfortunate husband. Such moods can veer between mild irritation and outright anger, and sometimes a woman may say really hurtful things that afterwards she deeply regrets. How comforting it is for her to know that her husband realizes that she does not mean it; that it is only because she loves him that he gets the full force of her emotional fragility.

Lethargy, vagueness, lack of concentration – these are among the effects of hormonal change that can affect a woman during pregnancy. There is nothing she can do about any of them when they descend on her. The more she tries to fight them, the worse they get. The more guilty she feels about the way she is behaving, the greater the tension and so a vicious circle is built up.

## ANTE-NATAL DEPRESSION

Another emotional problem that can occur in pregnancy is depression. We hear quite a lot about the post-natal 'maternity blues', but ante-natal depression is seldom mentioned. Few women go through a pregnancy, however, without encountering days when they feel depressed about the whole prospect of having a baby. Depression is a bit more than just feeling rather low: in pregnancy it tends to be a reaction to the woman's feelings of anxiety about what is happening to her in the whole process of reproduction.

Well-meaning friends and relations may not always make the situation easier when they show their enthusiasm and excitement over the expected birth: 'Aren't you excited?' 'You must be feeling so happy.' 'It's the most wonderful time in your life, waiting for your first baby.' They expect to find her knitting bootees and jackets and generally exuding an aura of radiant happiness as she prepares for the 'great event'. The fact that at this particular moment she is not excited, not knitting, not even wanting the baby, and not feeling radiantly happy, can make her feel guilty, and so actually increase her depression.

During the thirty years that I have been giving ante-natal classes, the number of girls who have wept on my shoulder because they were not feeling maternal and not looking forward to the birth of their babies is beyond' counting. One word of understanding and comfort, and an acknowledgement that, from time to time, such an experience is common to the majority of pregnant women, makes all the difference. To know that she is normal, that she is no different from other people, sets her mind at rest. But too often we tend to keep our fears and worries to ourselves, especially if we think they are not normal. To do this always exacerbates them. Women must be encouraged to discuss their problems and worries and to realize that they are reacting in a very normal way to pregnancy.

As her husband, and the father of the child she is expecting, you are able to give your wife this comfort and confidence better than anyone else – better than all the doctors, midwives and medical specialists in the world. Once she knows that you understand her feelings and the reasons for them, she will stop being afraid to discuss her changing emotions. And the more she can talk about her feelings, fears and anxieties, as well as her hopes and happiness, the better it will be for both of you.

## SHARING EMOTIONS

Pregnancy is a time of waiting, and waiting is seldom easy. It should also be a time of sharing: sharing the positive and negative emotions that will be intricately linked during the nine months leading up to the birth of the baby. It must never be thought that pregnancy is a period of nothing but tears and difficulties – far from it. Yet it is only human nature to accept the happy times without question, as if they were our right, and we are not

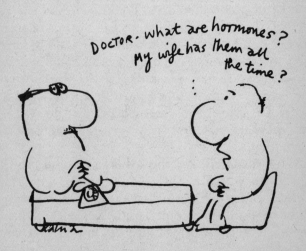

always as grateful for them as we ought to be. When the low moments and difficult situations present themselves, we all too easily allow them to predominate and make us forget the good things that we enjoy. But they are only part of the whole. Life is a jig-saw of good and bad; happy and unhappy; easy and difficult. We have to try to accept and learn from all the pieces as they fit into the pattern of our lives. During pregnancy, by sharing and understanding the fluctuating moods, a man and woman can begin to adapt together to the great change that is coming into their lives with the birth of their child.

# 2

# Sex during Pregnancy

The emotional changes in a pregnant woman can sometimes include a loss of libido, which is simply a term for our emotional drives towards physical love-making. Yes, the hormones are responsible for that as well. A lack of desire for sexual intercourse can at times cause unhappiness and place a strain on a relationship. The idea that his wife does not love him any more, or that she is becoming so preoccupied with the future baby that she has lost her interest in sex, can, quite naturally, make a man feel rejected, and sometimes a little jealous. This in turn will react on the woman, and so an unhappy, tense situation will arise and keep reinforcing itself. It is essential for the man and woman alike to understand that any apparent frigidity is, in such cases, beyond the woman's control. There is no magic button that she can press and instantaneously be filled with a great desire to make love. It is well known that if there are any sexual problems between a man and woman, tension on the part of either partner aggravates the difficulty.

FEAR NOT...

If a woman worries and feels guilty over her lack

of sexual desire it will only exacerbate the situation. She may feel the change that has occurred in her sexual drive will never reverse itself and come back to normal; that a happy sex life is over for ever. If she keeps these anxieties to herself they can grow out of all proportion. If these circumstances occur man and woman must content themselves with blaming the hormones again. The hormonal action is subtle and inevitable, and all the willing and wishing in the world will not change it, but it is not something that is going to last for ever.

Men can also sometimes find that their libido is affected during their wife's pregnancy. It may be a fear of hurting the wife while she seems so vulnerable; or of harming the baby in the womb; or of precipitating labour ahead of time. Such thoughts can interfere with a man's enjoyment of sex quite profoundly. Now it may be he who is the one to feel responsible for withholding the pleasures of a satisfying sexual relationship, and therefore precipitates the cycle of tensions and misunderstandings. By realizing the possibility of these problems, and understanding the reasons for them, by accepting them and discussing them, you can enrich the relationship.

The give and take of marriage will inevitably encounter some new, unfamiliar hurdles during pregnancy, especially if it is the first one. We must be careful not to approach any of these problems with a negative attitude, and so allow them to get out of proportion and become self-defeating and a cause of trouble. Rather they should be made an opportunity to surmount difficulties, and by so doing, create a greater depth and closeness in the inter-personal relationship between husband and wife.

We do not, however, need to create difficulties where none exist. In very many cases there will be no change in the intensity of sexual desire. Sometimes it can even increase, and for some couples pregnancy provides a time when inter-course can be enjoyed without any of the bothers of contraception or the fear of becoming pregnant unintentionally, and then such a sense of freedom allows for uninhibited enjoyment in love-making.

## 'GOOD MANNERS' IN LOVE-MAKING

There are, on the other hand, certain consider-ations that every amorous husband should keep in mind during his wife's pregnancy. We might perhaps call this simply a question of 'good manners'. Love-making should be gentle, especi-ally during the first month and the last three months. Your wife's breasts may become very tender, and as her abdomen enlarges and the baby creates pressures, this can cause great discomfort. The best position for intercourse can be found by experiment, e.g. a side position.

In fact in a straightforward pregnancy, inter-course may be continued up to the time of labour, and there are no factual reasons behind any of the old wives' tales that it should not take place after such and such a stage. On the other hand there may

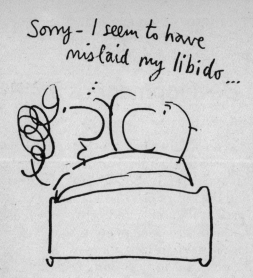

Sorry - I seem to have mislaid my libido...

be medical reasons why intercourse is inadvisable at certain times. If your wife has previously had a miscarriage it is essential that she should discuss this question with her doctor. Usually she will be advised not to have intercourse during the first three months, and especially not at the time when her first three periods would have been due.

Again, *any* bleeding during pregnancy at any stage should be taken as a warning against intercourse. If this occurs, your wife should get in touch with her doctor *at once* and he will advise when intercourse may be resumed. But the fact that intercourse may not be allowed does not mean that all love-making has to be forbidden. There are, after all, plenty of ways of expressing love that do not involve the complete sexual act.

# 3

# The Development of the Baby

There is no doubt that the sense of sharing, of looking forward together, is all the greater the more the man understands about the development of the baby and the future process of labour. For so many years pregnancy and childbirth were taboo subjects, not to be discussed in polite society. It was not considered 'nice' to talk about such things. Girls were brought up in horrifying ignorance of what should be such an important function in their lives – and boys even more so. Pregnancy and childbirth had 'nothing to do' with men. It was 'woman's work'. The man must be excluded. All this meant that a husband could feel very isolated during his wife's pregnancy, very much apart from the whole proceedings. Such an exaggerated sense of aloneness and anxiety of course affected both partners. This state of affairs has changed greatly in recent years, but men still often feel anxious during this time; they feel apart and cut off from what is happening.

## FATHER'S WORRIES

The expectant father naturally feels a great sense of responsibility towards the woman and his unborn child, but his role as a male has conditioned him to keep his anxieties to himself. Unexpressed fears may therefore increase out of all proportion and cause considerable problems. Some men suffer from insomnia. In others, digestive disturbances and skin rashes may be attributed directly to emotional stress over the wife's pregnancy. Stress of this nature is usually a result of ignorance and a consequent unconscious fear; and of childbirth having been dramatized too often over the years as 'something a woman has to go through'.

One man came to one of my Fathers' Evenings

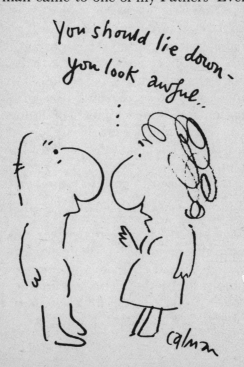

very reluctantly. His wife had warned me that he was extremely nervous. 'He just doesn't want to know,' she said. For several weeks he had been suffering from a very irritating rash that had not responded to treatment; his doctor called it his 'pregnancy rash'. As he left the Fathers' Evening he said to me: 'I feel as if a burden's been lifted now that I understand the whole procedure. What a miracle it all is.' Two days later his rash had disappeared! Such is the interaction between mind, emotion and body.

The conception, development and birth of a baby *is* a miracle, of course, and it is sad to think that so many thousands of couples still go through pregnancy and approach the important milestone of birth with fear, sometimes even with dread. Most men today have learned some rudimentary biology at school and so understand the principles of conception and the development of the foetus. Few, however, give much thought to the continuing miracle that is going on in a woman's body as her pregnancy progresses.

We do not need to go into too much technical detail in this book about the development of the baby. For those who are interested, there are some excellent books available that cover this subject. But a certain amount of basic knowledge is essential in helping to make the fact of pregnancy more acceptable for both the man and the woman. Moreover it can become an even more exciting time if you do know what is going on.

## WHAT HAPPENS IN THE WOMB?

The uterus, the medical term for the womb, is a pear-shaped organ situated in the pelvic cavity, and it measures approximately two by four inches. It is made up almost entirely of special muscle fibres that have an amazing capacity for stretching. Many women wonder how such a small organ will ever be able to stretch enough to accommodate a full-term baby that can weigh anything between six and ten pounds. 'I wake up in the night in a cold sweat, frightened that I'm going to split.' Only a few girls would openly express such a fear; most are afraid that people will think them stupid, so they keep it to themselves – which only exaggerates the fear. But the uterus is able to stretch as much as the growing baby demands.

From the upper part of the uterus, at the outer corners, there extends into the pelvic cavity a pair of ducts called Fallopian tubes. The outer ends of the tubes broaden into what are called fimbriae. These are finger-like processes that set up a continuous suction movement. Just behind the fimbriae, in the pelvic cavity, are the ovaries, one on each side of the body, in which the ova, or female cells, are produced and mature.

The maturing of an ovum, with which the menstrual cycle is connected, is highly complicated and results in the process known as ovulation. A ripe ovum is expelled once a month into the pelvic cavity, where it is drawn into the Fallopian tube by the suction of the fimbriae. It is then moved along the tube and down into the body of the uterus. An unfertilized ovum disintegrates as a matter of course and is excreted, along with the lining of the womb, during the menstrual period. As soon as the period is over, hormonal activity causes the lining of the womb to be prepared again for a possible conception. During menstruation the next ovum is maturing (one each month from alternate ovaries), leading to ovulation again two weeks later; and so the cycle repeats itself.

During intercourse sperms are ejaculated into the vagina. They then travel up through the cervical canal into the uterus and along the Fallopian tubes. Conception usually occurs towards the fimbriated end of the tube, and it happens at the moment when one sperm penetrates an ovum. A new cell is then formed and a new life has been started. The 'blueprint' of the future baby – its sex and all the genetic traits, such as the colour of hair and eyes, the shape of ears and nose – have been laid down. A sperm is microscopic, an ovum is approximately the size of a grain of sand; yet in the course of forty weeks a baby weighing an average of seven and a half pounds will develop – a human being ready to start a life of his own, with all the intricate functioning that goes to make up the species known as *Homo sapiens*.

## WHAT HAPPENS AFTER CONCEPTION?

Once conception has occurred the embryo moves along the Fallopian tube into the body of the uterus. By now it will have divided and subdivided

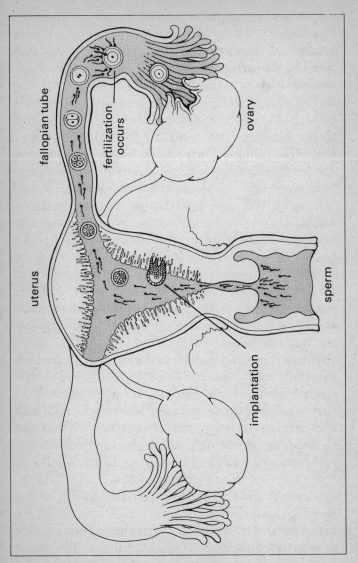

Fig. 1 Fertilization and implantation.

to become a group of cells, and this group implants itself into the lining of the uterus. The implantation is nearly always at the upper part of the uterus, and is the point at which the placenta or 'after-birth' will develop.

The placenta is a very complex organ, formed by an intricate network of blood vessels and connected to the baby via the umbilical cord. The placenta and the umbilical cord thus make the link between mother and baby. It is the activity of the placenta and the flow of blood through the cord that nourishes and develops the baby throughout its foetal stage of development. The placenta grows with the foetus until at term – the time when the baby is due to be born – it will be round, some six to seven inches in diameter and about one and a half inches thick, and approximately one-sixth of the baby's weight. As is implied by its familiar name, the afterbirth will eventually be delivered after the birth of the baby.

From the moment of conception development is rapid. At four weeks the foetus would be just visible to the naked eye. At six weeks it is less than half an inch long, but the spinal cord has been formed and the internal organs and circulatory system are developing. Arm buds and leg buds are forming, and the eyes, nose and mouth are all taking shape.

By the end of ten weeks most of the organs are completely formed, the heart is beating, the baby is moving – though the mother will not as yet be aware of any movement. The length of the foetus is now approximately two inches and it weighs about an ounce.

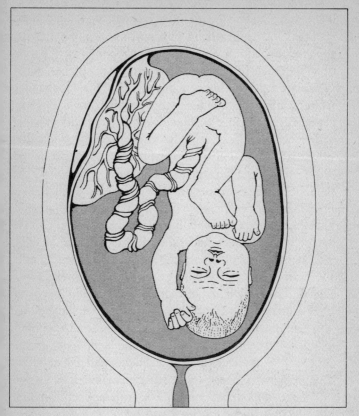

Fig. 2   Placenta, umbilical cord and baby.

By the end of the fourteenth week, or three and a half months, the baby is completely formed. He is about four inches long. The genitals have developed to a point where the sex of the baby can be determined. The various body systems are beginning to function.

The mother will usually start to be aware of the

baby moving between the sixteenth and twentieth weeks. On the question of foetal movement during pregnancy, the point that there are varying degrees of movement needs some stressing, as this can cause great anxiety to expectant mothers. If the husband understands this he can give his wife some welcome reassurance. Some babies move more than others. Some women feel hardly any movement, while others are kicked about continuously. The situation varies from one woman to another.

All women tend to feel anxiety about the normality of their unborn baby. They worry about whether it is going to have the normal quota of arms, legs, fingers, toes and so on. Your own wife will be no exception. If the baby moves very little she will imagine that it has no arms and legs to move about. If it kicks a great deal she will worry that it may have too many arms and legs! And worry she will, make no mistake about it; and as the day for delivery comes closer, she will worry even more. The burden of her anxiety will be enormously relieved, however, if she can talk to you about her seemingly irrational fears and be confident of your sympathetic understanding.

One other point that can cause your wife alarm as pregnancy progresses is the extent to which she is showing her pregnancy. This depends largely on the length of her waist and the way the baby is lying. I have known some long-waisted women who have, at full term, still barely shown their pregnancy. Others who are short-waisted have, at six months, had it suggested to them by well-meaning friends that perhaps they are in for twins!

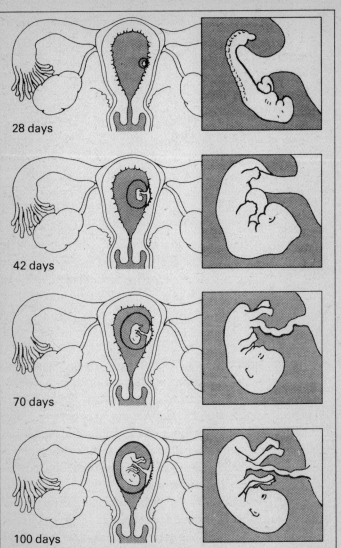

28 days

42 days

70 days

100 days

Fig. 3   Development of the baby.

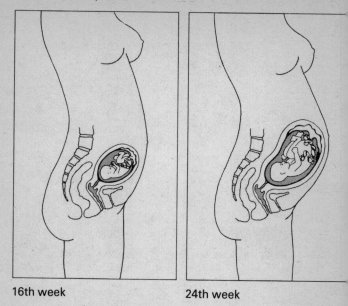

16th week                    24th week

Fig. 4   Development of the baby (continued).

Friends and relatives can, by unthinking remarks, cause more hurt and anxiety than they can possibly realize. It is difficult to stop them from indulging in the happy pastimes of diagnosing and giving good advice, but if the differences that can occur in degrees of foetal movement and evidence of pregnancy are understood, heartache and anxiety will be kept to the minimum.

From six months on the prime purpose of development is size and maturity. The closer to term a baby is, the better. During the last two months of pregnancy a baby almost doubles its

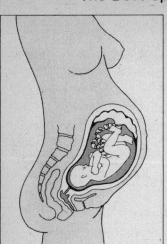
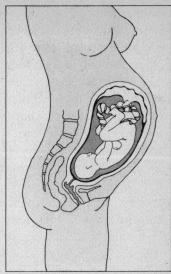

32nd week                34th-36th week

Fig. 5   Development of the baby (continued).

weight, and the final and important factors of maturation occur. It is, however, an old wives' tale, and one that has no truth in it whatsoever, that says that a baby born at seven months is more likely to survive than one born at eight months.

## ENCOURAGING LABOUR TO START

Sometimes there may be obstetrical reasons for inducing labour a little early. If, for instance, a doctor suspects that placental activity is diminishing, certain tests will be done to find out whether this is indeed happening. If it is, labour may be induced to ensure that the baby is born before any harmful effects develop from lack of nourishment owing to a faulty functioning of the placenta. Most pregnancies progress normally without any such problems arising but we must face facts and accept that sometimes difficulties do occur. Today we can be very grateful for the medical expertise which, by means of special blood tests, ultrasound scanning and other techniques, can diagnose problems relating to either the mother or the baby and initiate the necessary treatment without delay.

By the end of the thirty-sixth week, or eighth month, the baby is almost fully mature. Before he is born he will be swallowing, urinating and establishing the digestive process. In fact he is preparing for the momentous event of his birth, and of his becoming a separated individual, and his survival will be dependent on the successful co-ordination of all the complex systems in his body.

## TOLERATING THE INCONVENIENCES

It is at about the thirty-sixth week, or perhaps a little earlier, that the baby 'drops', and the head becomes engaged into the pelvic cavity as it gets ready for delivery. This engaging of the head is usually a gradual process. As the days go by a woman becomes aware that the restriction on her breathing has eased slightly. She feels a little more space under her ribs, though this relief is counter-acted by an increasing pressure on her bladder as the baby's head presses lower and lower into the pelvis. Sometimes it is very difficult for the poor husband to appreciate what the effects of this pressure lead to. Every fifteen minutes his wife wants to find a 'loo'. It seems to him impossible that she could want to go so often, and it is always at an inconvenient time, or in an impossibly inconvenient place. But babies, both *in utero* and after they are born, are no respecters of time or place, and in the last weeks before delivery they certainly crack the whip as far as these uncontrollable physiological needs of their mothers are concerned.

The physical discomforts of pregnancy do indeed require some special considerations at times. During the first three months your wife's life can be made miserable by fatigue and nausea. 'Morning sickness' is a very well known problem of early

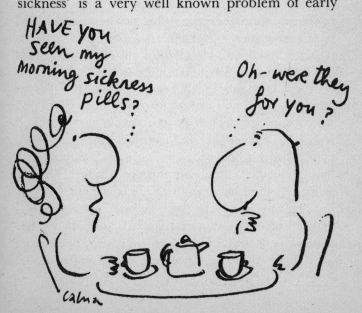

pregnancy, but the unbelievable sleepiness which can overcome women is not so well recognized. Both these symptoms usually clear up after the third month, but can return during the last two months, and many women are surprised and discomfited to find nausea and vomiting once more a problem. Later on, her increasing weight makes movement more difficult. She may suffer from backache and may sometimes have difficulty in walking. These changes may cause irritation, for they interfere with the normal flow of life. At this point one needs to stop and think of the reasons for them, and to realize that they are symptoms of the amazing processes involved in the development and birth of a new human being. Then it all falls into a proper perspective.

The stretching sensation that many women feel in the joint between the pubic bones, and the pain (the 'sciatic pain') that can go down the back of the leg and make walking so difficult, are the result of the loosening of the joints in the pelvis and pressure on the sciatic nerve. This loosening of the joints is nature's way of ensuring that there will be maximum space for a baby to emerge. Some women are more affected than others by this. Any expectant mother with sciatic pain should be seen by her doctor, and for some women it may reach a point when resting on a hard bed is essential. It is important to stress the need for rest, and to walk as little as possible if she suffers sciatic pain. When she does walk, a walking stick can be a great support and relieve the pressure on the sciatic nerve. Some women feel very self-conscious about using a walking stick, but it is better to use one and relieve the strain than to hobble around increasing the condition as well as the pain. So much stress is put on the need for exercise during pregnancy, and helpful friends and relatives suggest the best treatment is to 'take more exercise my dear, to make the muscles more supple'. Taking exercise is indeed very beneficial, but it is the worst thing a woman can do if she is afflicted by this sacro-iliac problem.

Due to hormonal change there is an increase of the mucous secretions in the body during pregnancy, and this is the cause of the nasal catarrh which so many women experience. Sometimes it reaches a point where breathing through the nose becomes difficult and sometimes impossible. It is also the cause of women snoring when they are pregnant. Many girls have said to me, 'My husband complains that I'm snoring. What can I do about it?'. There is nothing she can do. It is advisable for her to sleep with her head as high as is comfortable and perhaps it is sensible for her husband to wear ear-plugs! As soon as pregnancy is over she will return to her silent sleeping habits!

As the last few weeks of pregnancy are reached signs and symptoms occur that are indications of the onset of labour approaching. Mucus vaginal discharge can become heavier, and a woman usually begins to feel regular contractions, which are the sign of increasing hormonal activity; the cervix is beginning to thin and the build-up to the start of labour is under way.

During the last few weeks of pregnancy, as the baby grows bigger and drops lower, the movements are usually no longer felt as strongly as before. There is, quite simply, not so much space in which the baby can move around. But it is untrue to say that a baby becomes completely still. He will, in fact, go on moving throughout labour, though the movements become far less noticeable to the mother.

## KEEPING THE DOCTOR INFORMED

What has been said above deals with a normal 'head-first' delivery. There are, however instances where something has occurred which may require special treatment, even perhaps a Caesarean operation and this is dealt with later in Chapter 10. The importance, at this point, is stressed of the mother-to-be being under her doctor's care and observation regularly, as soon as conception is known. This means that if any minor or even more serious problems should develop they can be noted and either corrected or arrangements made for them to be dealt with by the numerous methods of modern medical science available.

# 4

# The Importance of Breathing Techniques

Your wife should ask her doctor about ante-natal clinics in your area. Here she will be able to find out what ante-natal classes are available. She should be encouraged to attend these classes so that she can learn about the relaxation and breathing techniques that will help her through labour when the time comes.

About three weeks before her 'estimated date of confinement', she should have been given all the information about the process of childbirth so that she will go into labour with a full understanding of what is about to happen and with a knowledge of what she can do to help herself. A positive attitude of confidence in herself and in her obstetrical team is the most effective weapon that any woman can possess to carry her through labour.

DOING THE EXERCISES

Your wife's breathing exercises may seem to you to be among the more eccentric things that she brings home to do after her ante-natal classes. But whether or not you are planning to sit with your wife during labour, it is important for you to know about the breathing techniques that she is being taught. Then if you are going to be there you will understand what she is doing, and why she is doing it; otherwise it can be most alarming for the uninitiated to hear a woman start to breathe in what sounds like a very strange fashion. If you are there you will be able to encourage her and remind her if she forgets her breathing exercises. If you are not going to be there, the very fact that you understand the principle underlying the breathing will give you a sense of confidence in knowing that your wife has something to do that can afford her great and genuine help during labour. Knowing this will relieve you of much anxiety.

For these reasons I suggest it can be very useful for you, as her husband, to learn the breathing yourself. It will help *you* to have the practical knowledge, and it will help *her* to be encouraged to practise it and to feel that it is a shared effort. Pregnancy can be a lonely road for both man and woman, and practising together can help to create a greater sense of understanding and sharing.

The breathing techniques taught will differ somewhat from one class to another. I am going to explain here the breathing that I have found to be most useful during labour. It is essential that the breathing used in labour should be kept as simple and effortless as possible, and although I use the word 'level' for want of a better one, there should be no rigidity about it.

FIRST LEVEL

Breathe *out* and *in*, gently and rhythmically, *emphasizing slightly the outward breath*. The amount of breath inhaled will be in the same proportion as that exhaled, and it may make it easier if one thinks of *letting* the breath come in rather than actively taking a breath in. This gentle emphasis on the outward breath helps to stop a woman from holding her breath during a labour contraction, and also prevents her from gasping in her breath – which can lead to overbreathing and 'hyper-ventilation'.

*Breathe with the lips separated.* I do not advocate breathing with the mouth wide open. In fact it is better not to think in terms of breathing through

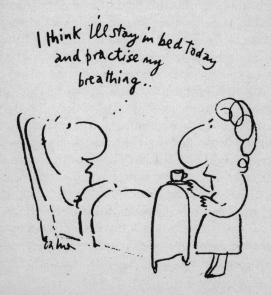

I think I'll stay in bed today and practise my breathing..

the nose or mouth, but rather of breathing with the lips not completely closed, and this will allow the breathing to change automatically as circumstances demand.

*Do not breathe out too deeply*. If she breathes out too deeply, she will also breathe in too deeply, and it is important that she should not breathe down into her abdomen. If the breath is drawn in too deeply, she will be breathing down into the pain and not keeping on top of it, which is the principle behind the technique.

*The breathing must never be forced*. She should breathe in a way that is comfortable for her, just remembering the three points emphasized above. The really important aspect of the breathing is her concentration on it. When she practises the breathing, she should listen to it, be aware of herself breathing. She should do it with a sense of purpose, with an attitude that says: 'I am doing it'; it should not be just happening. It is far better to do three or four breaths with complete attention than to carry on breathing for a minute while thinking of something else.

In fact it is important, when practising, not to continue breathing in this way for longer than thirty seconds. For it is an abnormal way in which to breathe when there is no energy expenditure to warrant it, and if it is continued for too long it can lead to breathlessness or dizziness. If, while practising, breathlessness or dizziness do occur, it is a sign that she is breathing with too much effort or is continuing for too long. During her labour there will be a reason for doing it: she will concentrate on keeping above pain, and she will find that she will be able to continue for as long as the need demands.

## SECOND LEVEL - SHALLOWER

Start with two or three breaths of the first level, and then gradually make the breathing a little shallower and quicker, letting it rise as far as is comfortable; then bring it down again, slower and deeper, but always emphasizing gently the out-ward breath. Everyone has a different rhythm of breathing and it is *very* important that no one should try to force their breathing too far out of its norm. I have taught many women whose normal rhythm of breathing was so slow that it was too difficult for them to change it to a shallow level. But in labour it fitted into its appropriate pattern without difficulty.

## THIRD LEVEL - HUFFING AND PUFFING

This third way of breathing I call 'huffing and puffing'. At first sight (or sound!) it may seem slightly insane, but it can be a very useful weapon during labour. It is a variation of shallow breathing; two shallow breaths, OUT-in, OUT-in, BLOW-in, BLOW-in. The BLOW is what one would do when blowing out a match. Many people, who normally breathe slowly and who cannot manage the shallow level, find that huffing and puffing comes quite easily.

These three levels of breathing should be practised several times a day. It is important that your wife does not make a fetish of it and become tense about it in her efforts to get it 'right'. She should simply practise taking her attention off whatever she is doing at a given moment and concentrating on the breathing at whichever level she chooses. If she does this a few times a day, using the different levels, she will find in quite a short time that it becomes automatic.

## THE APPLICATION OF BREATHING TECHNIQUES

How then, will your wife apply this breathing during her actual labour?

Labour contractions are like waves: they start, build to a peak, level out at that peak for a certain time and then fade. In the very early part of labour, the wave is not very high and the contraction does not last long (perhaps 15 or 20 seconds) and any pain is negligible. As the first stage of labour progresses, the contractions will become stronger and the pain increases as they build to their peak more quickly and last longer. Just before full dilatation of the cervix is achieved, the contractions can be coming once every two minutes and lasting nearly two minutes. At this point of labour it can seem to a woman that there is no space between them. It is nearly always the most difficult part of labour, but it will help her enormously if she knows that these long, strong, almost continuous contractions mean that the end is in sight. Again her positive attitude will be her great strength.

To show what a difference the breathing will make for your wife in labour, and how its rhythm will change, it is interesting to try a simple experiment. Allow someone to pinch you. Resist what is being done by tensing up against it, and be aware of the pain that you are feeling. Now let the person pinch you again, but this time do not tense up and resist it. Focus your attention on some object and breathe at it with the first level of breathing, making your attention follow along the line of your breath towards the object. I am sure you will notice that the pain will be less.

Next let the person pinch you, starting fairly gently and gradually increasing the strength. Breathe 'above' the pain, as it were, allowing your breathing to change as the increased pain demands. You will find that the rhythm of your breathing will alter automatically with the increase in the pain stimulus. Women are often very anxious that when it comes to labour, they will not know at which point to vary the rhythm of their breathing. This simple experiment usually convinces them of how automatic the change will be so long as they *keep breathing*, always gently emphasizing the outward breath.

This principle remains true wherever the pain is and whatever sort of physical pain is involved. If attention can be diverted from the point of pain by some sort of distraction, the pain threshold is raised and the person involved becomes less conscious of the pain stimulus. It is for this reason that it is so vital for a woman to concentrate absolutely on her breathing during a contraction. This is not always easy for her.

We are conditioned from early childhood to conform to rules of social politeness and to speak when spoken to. In labour, all such rules must be abandoned. Nothing and no one must be allowed to interfere with the mother-to-be's concentration. Here again you will be able to help, if you do happen to be with her during labour. So many women have mentioned to me afterwards how helpful it was to have their husbands with them for this reason. As one girl said: 'He acted as a buffer between me and the staff. If anyone spoke to me during a contraction, he was there to answer for me and to explain that I just couldn't talk at that moment. He helped me keep my concentration in the middle of everything going on around me.'

Doctors and nurses do not mean to interrupt, but sometimes they speak to a woman before they realize that she is in the middle of a contraction. Without someone there who understands the situation to remind her, the reflex to be polite, built in over the years, may easily make her respond – and lose her concentration.

To suppose that relaxing and breathing are guaranteed to make labour painless is, of course, ridiculous. It would be very wrong even to suggest such a possibility. If this idea is instilled into a woman's mind, and subsequently during labour she experiences what she feels to be considerable pain, the resulting effects can be traumatic indeed. She will feel badly let down, that she herself has failed in some way, and an unhappy situation will be created that may cause great problems and unnecessary anxieties during any future pregnancy.

The purpose of the breathing techniques is to give a woman something constructive to do in labour that will help to distract her attention away from the pain. Without such a technique she can feel helpless in a situation that she does not understand, and the inevitable tension that follows will exacerbate the pain.

Most women find it helpful if they do their breathing during a contraction with their eyes open and focussing their attention on an object some distance away – say a picture, a spot on the wall or a

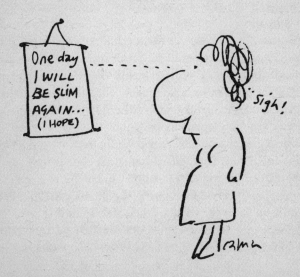

bowl of flowers. This helps to hold their attention away from the pain. There is no rigid rule about this, and some women prefer to keep their eyes closed. But for the majority, breathing with their eyes open helps them to remain as relaxed as possible and to maintain their concentration.

Anyone sitting with a woman in labour will find it easy to see if she is losing control of concentration and breathing. She will show signs of distress, and then it can help her immeasurably if you make her open her eyes and look at you. You can then lead her back into the breathing by doing it with her, and she will be able to follow you. As another girl told me: 'The only time I became submerged was when I closed my eyes. Then I felt I was right inside the pain. But my husband saved the situation. He almost shouted at me, "Open your eyes!" and breathed with me. Immediately I felt myself up on top again.'

Unless there is some obstetrical reason why she should be lying down in bed during the early stages – and if there is she will, of course, be told not to get up – it is better for a woman going into labour to keep moving around during the earlier hours, and to stay in an upright position during the contractions. Keeping busy will help her to pass the time, and standing up during a contraction will help labour to progress more quickly.

Many women find it comfortable to lean against a wall, or to bend over and support themselves on the back of a chair or on a bed end. It can be very disconcerting for a husband who does not understand the situation to see his wife suddenly droop against a wall with her mouth slightly open and an expressionless look on her face as she starts breathing into the distance. The one thing she does not want at that moment is a worried husband asking her what she is doing or whether she is all right. What she will need more than anything is a word of encouragement to keep breathing, a reminder that there is just this one contraction to deal with at this moment; and, afterwards, a quiet, 'Well done'.

## PROGRESS OF LABOUR

No one can prophesy exactly what any particular person's labour is going to be like, how it will start or how long it will last. Even once it has started, there is no way of knowing what pattern it will follow. Some labours progress more quickly than others. The length of labour depends to a great extent on the position of the baby, the woman's hormonal activity and the degree to which the cervix has been taken up before true labour has become established. I have known labours to last anything between two hours and thirty-six hours (between six and twelve hours is said to be the average for a first baby). First confinements are usually the longest; second and subsequent ones are generally much shorter.

Sometimes a labour can be overwhelmingly quick, which makes it difficult for the woman to keep up with the speed of her contractions.

Whatever the pattern of a labour, however, be it a short or a long one, it has to be accepted *as it is*. A woman cannot change the pattern of her labour; she can never will it to be different. But, by accepting it and taking the contractions one by one, she will always keep any difficulties to a minimum. It can help tremendously to remind a woman of this. If a labour is going very quickly, she could be wishing that it would slow down a little to let her get her breath back between contractions. If it is progressing slowly, she can become impatient and frustrated and wonder if it will ever end. If you remind her that it is not possible either to slow things up or hurry them along, it will bring her back to the reality of the situation; and this, in turn, will help her to accept it and concentrate on dealing with it, contraction by contraction.

With this basic knowledge you will be in a position to help when the moment comes – as come it will – when your wife goes into labour.

We have spoken of the husband helping, but of course it is not always possible for a husband to be there and some men do not want to be. Then, this advice may be helpful in guiding the mother as to what she may wish to ask for.

# 5

# Preparing for Labour

Meanwhile the preparations are going forward, both psychological and practical. During the last weeks of pregnancy the usual anxieties, especially those concerning the normality of the baby, will inevitably be to the fore. And, of course, no doctor will be able to alleviate these worries completely. They are there, and no woman goes through pregnancy without them. But how comforting it is for her to know that she is no different from the thousands of other pregnant women who are approaching the onset of labour.

She should never feel diffident about asking for advice. So often women are reluctant to telephone the hospital or doctor for fear of being thought over-anxious or stupid, but it is always better to err on the side of caution and to seek advice that is there for the asking. In fact if she feels concern over anything in particular at any time during pregnancy, she should have no hesitation in telling her doctor or midwife. Too often a woman will not mention what is worrying her, and as we know, unexpressed fears can soon grow out of all proportion.

TESTS

Another thing that can happen is that during visits to the ante-natal clinic doctors or midwives casually use technical terms that, because they are not understood by the woman, are immediately interpreted in her mind as meaning that something is going wrong. Tests may be carried out to ensure that pregnancy is progressing normally and that the baby is developing well. Ultrasound examinations, a particular twenty-four hour urine test, and certain blood tests are common procedures which are used very frequently. For the doctor and midwife these are everyday occurrences, but for the pregnant woman they may appear to be indications that something is not quite normal. If only she could simply ask at such moments: 'What does that mean? Please tell me, or I shall worry.' In most cases the problem would then quickly be sorted out. But she may be shy about doing so, about revealing what she feels to be her ignorance, and so she takes the worry home with her.

Doctors and midwives are busy people. They work under great pressure and do not always realize the anxieties that may be created by inadvertent remarks. For them, specialized medical terms are in ordinary, everyday use. It is difficult for them to remember that their patients may have no understanding of these terms. A gentle reminder of this fact, and a question about exactly what is meant, will almost certainly bring a simple explanation. Should your wife be nervous about asking, however, and should a worry persist, I suggest that you, as her husband, do the asking for her, mentioning her reluctance to speak of it and explaining the tension that the unsolved problem is causing.

Assure your wife in advance of labour itself that, if she wishes, you will act as spokesman when that time comes so that she can share even the tiniest worry straight away knowing you can swiftly call for the answer for her.

Your wife will have been given a list of things that she should have ready to take into hospital with her or available in the house if it is to be a home confinement. It is important that the lists should be completed in good time. No one can say exactly when labour will begin. It can start at any time once she is within two weeks of the 'estimated date of confinement'; it can likewise be at any time during the two weeks following the estimated date.

# PART II

# LABOUR

# 6

# The Onset of Labour

The onset of labour is usually easily recognizable, and it can start in one of three ways: a) with contractions (which are quite distinct from the mild contractions that occur throughout pregnancy); b) with a 'show' of mucus and blood; or c) with the rupture of the membranes – the 'breaking of the waters'.

## 'FALSE LABOUR'

Labour is simply an extension of pregnancy. During the last few weeks there will be gradual changes in hormonal activity that affect the muscle action of the uterus. It is this that can cause the false alarms (the so-called 'false labour') experienced by so many women. They feel contractions: a regular, rhythmic tightening in the abdomen. Sometimes these contractions can come and go regularly, every ten minutes for two or three hours, before they suddenly stop. Rushing into hospital, only to be told to go home again because this is not yet proper labour, can leave the wife and everyone else with a great feeling of anticlimax and demoralisation. Labour cannot be said to have got properly under way until the contractions change in character and become stronger and last longer.

One girl whom I had taught had contractions for twenty-seven hours before they began to build up and become painful. They started one evening. When she went to bed she took a mild sedative prescribed by her doctor and slept well, but every time she woke up the contractions were still coming and going as before. The next day she went about things quite normally, and even spent the afternoon at the cinema, still aware of the regular contractions, but not worrying about them as they remained the same in character, lasting only about twenty seconds at a time and causing no pain. Eventually, she noticed a change: they had begun to become painful and were lasting longer; she had to start doing the breathing she had learned. Eight hours later her son was born. As she told me afterwards: 'If I hadn't understood the whole process I'd have rushed into hospital as soon as the contractions started, and I'd have said afterwards that it had been a thirty-five-hour labour.' But in fact she had an eight-hour labour, and because she had not become too involved too soon, had not watched the clock and counted hours, her morale had remained high; and after the baby was born she felt well and unfatigued.

It is only natural for a man to feel extremely nervous over any delay in getting his wife to hospital. In his horrified imagination he sees her suddenly producing the baby on the kitchen floor! But rushing to hospital in a panic helps no one, least of all the woman herself. Rather it can help a great deal if she keeps herself busy doing odd jobs, and walking about. If she is upright during a contraction the force of gravity helps the descent of the baby towards the birth canal. A comfortable position for her can be leaning against a wall or supporting herself by bending over and holding on to a chair. The one thing she should never do during this onset stage is to sit and wait for the next contraction to start. That can be very demoralising. And provided the membranes have not ruptured a warm bath can be very relaxing and relieving to any pain.

## 'BREAKING OF THE WATERS'

There is in fact no need for immediate concern if the membranes rupture, though it can be an embarrassing inconvenience. Water may be felt trickling involuntarily down the legs, or it may suddenly gush out in something of a torrent! This can be very alarming for a woman who has not been forewarned of the possibility; and alarming, too, for her husband, if he happens to be there at the time.

If the membranes do rupture your wife *must* inform whoever is responsible for her – doctor, midwife or hospital – and then be patient and wait for labour to begin. If she is having the baby in hospital, she will almost certainly be told to come in. If she is having a home delivery the midwife will need to know so that she can visit her patient and make all the necessary preparations.

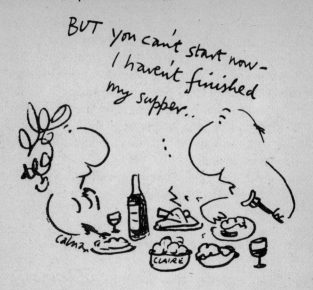

There may be a few hours' delay before true labour starts. It is most important to keep time in its proper perspective. Nothing can be more demoralising in labour than clock-watching, and it is a wise woman who does not become involved too soon – and a wise husband who refrains from panic and from creating needless anxieties.

## THE 'SHOW'

The same principle over the rupturing of the membranes also applies to the 'show' – the loss of the mucus plug that forms in the cervical canal during pregnancy. The 'show' is usually stained with a little blood and may be taken as an indication that the cervix is starting to undergo its necessary change before labour begins. It is therefore a common sign that the onset of labour will probably not be long delayed, and is nothing to feel concerned about but if a woman loses more blood than she would consider as 'staining', she should report it to the doctor or hospital.

## CONTRACTIONS WHEN LABOUR STARTS

The general rule is that we do not say that labour has started simply because some mild, painless contractions are being felt; or because the membranes have ruptured; or because a 'show' of mucus and blood has appeared. On the question of exactly when a woman should go into hospital, provided the membranes have not ruptured, I suggest she should go in as soon as the contractions become stronger, start to change in character and last longer. If they cause sufficient pain to make her need to concentrate on her breathing, she should certainly go in. And if she feels nervous, and *wants* to go in, then it is wise for her to do so. If she is at all anxious, even if the contractions are very mild, it is much better for her to go in so that she can be examined and reassured. If it is not yet true labour, there is no shame in coming home again, but staying at home as anxieties and tensions mount is not going to do anyone any good.

# 7

# The First Stage of Labour

Once true labour has begun it is the culmination of months of waiting. It is important to understand as much as possible about the process of labour. Without such understanding it can be very frightening, both for the woman who is going through it and for the man, who will perhaps be pacing the corridor in traditional style, or waiting anxiously for news at home or in his office, or sitting by the bed, feeling helpless and wishing there was something he could be getting on with to assist his wife.

Fear through ignorance has been the cause of so much unhappiness in the past. Not so long ago all women approached their confinements conditioned to the idea that labour was an ordeal they had to suffer; that there was nothing they could do to help themselves and they would just have to bear it as best they could. The wonder and beauty of childbirth were seldom talked about. I can vouch for this from my own experience, having been brought up in an age in which pregnancy and childbirth were shrouded in secrecy. If ever these subjects were mentioned, it was probably by someone saying: 'I hope she won't have too bad a time'; or: 'Poor dear, I'm afraid she had a terrible time'; or, to a child asking awkward questions, the sinister answer: 'You'll find out soon enough.' The power of suggestion can be very strong and it plays an important part in our lives. The continual frightening hints and innuendoes about what labour was like, gleaned from conversations, books and the cinema, built into me, as with the majority of girls, a fear of what would one day probably happen to me.

In due course I trained as a nurse, and during my obstetrical nursing I helped to deliver many women who had been conditioned as I had been. They came into labour afraid and tense and suffered, as I realized years later, quite unnecessarily. In due course my own turn came, and although I understood all about the procedure from the professional point of view, my personal attitude to it was completely negative. I was afraid of the pain that I thought was inevitable, and I went through my first labour feeling as helpless and unhappy as anyone else. There is no doubt that it has been this sense of helplessness, this negative attitude of 'it's being done to me and there's nothing I can do about it,' that has been so traumatic for so many women. The positive attitude of 'I am having a baby and I know what to do to help', with which a woman should approach labour, was submerged under a welter of negative suggestions, old wives' tales and the dramatization of childbirth as an ordeal a woman had to experience before she could achieve motherhood.

We must remember that every human being is

made up of mind, emotions and body. The three can never be separated, and what affects one will affect the others. If there is tension in the form of fear or anger at the emotional level, the body will immediately become tense too, and it is important to realize the significance of this where labour is concerned. When a woman goes into labour afraid and feeling helpless, tension will occur throughout her body. If she tenses up against pain, the pain will increase, and this, of course, increases the fear, which in turn increases the tension – and so the vicious circle is set in motion. This fear/tension/pain syndrome was at the root of the helpless, unhappy situation that confronted so many women in the past.

## BUILDING THE POSITIVE ATTITUDE

Even today, in a so-called 'permissive' age, we are far from being entirely free of the older prejudiced attitudes. Much can be altered, however, by instilling in a woman the confidence that comes from understanding the changes that occur during pregnancy, the mechanism of labour and the obstetrical procedures that may be used. Knowledge will dispel the fears causing the physical tension, and so break the fear/tension/pain syndrome. She will then be able to approach labour with the positive attitude which we have seen is so important – with confidence in herself as well as in the obstetrical team caring for her. Armed with this confidence and knowledge, even if her labour does not follow the average pattern, she will accept the obstetrical help she may need with gratitude and without fear, and will encounter no traumatic after-effects.

Once a man appreciates the logic of the fear/tension/pain syndrome, and understands the mechanism of labour, it will be a source of enormous help to his wife. The fact that he understands gives her a feeling of confidence, a sense of sharing with him in the job she has to do, whether or not he plans to be with her throughout labour. And for him, the bogey of childbirth and the fear of what his wife may be going to suffer will be relieved. Of course it cannot eliminate all anxiety. It would be foolish to suggest as much. But the natural worries that precede any event as important as childbirth can be balanced by a rational understanding of all the aspects involved.

## WHAT HAPPENS IN LABOUR?

First of all then, what exactly is happening as labour is taking place? It is all very well to say: 'A baby is being born.' How is this being accomplished? It comes about by a remarkable process of muscle action in the uterus (or womb). As has already been explained (page 29), the uterus is a pear-shaped organ. The larger part of it, in which the baby develops, is called the body, and the narrow neck of the uterus is called the cervix. The muscular structure of the uterus is very complicated, and we do not need to go into close anatomical detail to understand what is happening. We do not, in fact, need to do more than deal with just two sets of muscles: longitudinal muscles that run up and down the uterus, extending over the top of it, and horizontal, circular muscle fibres that are concentrated round the lower segment of the uterus. During the months of pregnancy these circular muscles remain tightened in order to keep the cervix closed and the foetus securely in the body of the womb where it can develop and reach maturity. Before the baby can be born, therefore, the cervix must be dilated; the door, so to speak, must be opened to allow the passage of the baby out of the uterus.

Opening the cervix is the objective of the first stage of labour. It is achieved by the contraction of the muscles that cover the body of the uterus. As a woman goes into labour and her contractions begin, each so-called pain is, in fact, caused by the long muscles contracting and gradually retracting the lower part of the womb, so taking up and stretching the cervix until, at the end of the first stage of labour, it is fully dilated. At the same time the uterus, which has expanded so remarkably to accommodate a fully developed foetus, is now contracting down again and will, by the time delivery is completed, be about the size of a large grapefruit. Hence there is a definite purpose in each contraction; they are, one by one, accomplishing the first important goal in the process of childbirth: the full dilatation of the cervix. This first stage of labour lasts from the onset of labour until the dilatation of the cervix is completed, and is usually the longest and most tedious part of the whole process.

But provided a woman realizes that each contraction is taking her one step closer to the birth of her baby; that there is a purpose to each of them; that each one is achieving something; then she can accept them with a positive attitude. And provided she has been to ante-natal classes and learned breathing and relaxing techniques, she will now be able to do something constructive to assist the muscle action of her uterus. She can, in other words, work with her uterus rather than being lead by fear and tension to fight against the inevitable.

It is difficult to describe where or how a woman will feel her contractions. This will depend to a large extent on the position of the baby in the uterus. Most women describe contractions as period-like pains felt low down in the abdomen, which sometimes extend round to the back. Some women feel contractions only in the lower part of the back, with no pain in the abdomen at all. I have even known a few women who have felt their contractions in their thighs. But wherever a woman feels them, the contractions will never cause a sudden, sharp spasm. There is always the building up to a peak and then the fading away.

## THE PROGRESSION OF THE FIRST STAGE

It may help to think of labour as a road going up a mountain, with the contractions as steps on the

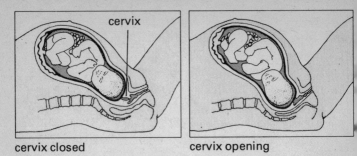

cervix

cervix closed

cervix opening

Fig. 6 Dilatation of the cervix.

road that become steeper the higher one climbs. As the contractions grow stronger, so the goal comes closer; one by one they are bringing a woman nearer to the birth of her baby. This idea of 'one by one' is vital. She will never have to deal with two at a time, nor with the same one twice. It is when a woman looks ahead in labour and wonders, 'How much longer is all this going on?' that she can become discouraged, and may possibly abandon her correct breathing.

This is the point where the help of a husband sitting with his wife during labour can be invaluable. He can remind her that *this one* contraction is the only one on which she has to concentrate, and that once it is over it will have gone into the past and can never come again. It is impossible to overstress how important this sense of purpose is: the knowledge that the contractions are doing something positive, and that, one by one, they are carrying the mother-to-be towards her ultimate goal.

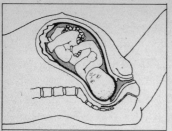
cervix half dilated

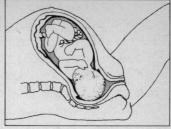
full dilatation

Dilation of the cervix (continued).

As a contraction starts, so a woman must start the breathing, the idea being that she will always breathe 'above' the contraction. Which of the three levels of breathing she uses will depend on the circumstances of the moment. If the contraction is not strong, and the wave is not 'high', she uses the lower, slower level of breathing. She breathes as slowly, deeply (without breathing deeply into the abdomen), rhythmically and effortlessly as the contraction will allow. As the contractions become stronger and the pain increases, so the breathing becomes shallower and faster to help her stay above it. The 'huffing and puffing' is the extra gear, so to speak, for any time when she feels that the other breathing is not quite carrying her. The difference in pattern of the huffing and puffing demands greater concentration and so helps to lift her attention that much more above the pain.

The change in her rhythm of breathing will occur automatically if a woman starts each contraction with the positive thought: 'Good, I know what I'm doing, I'm going with it.' You may think that I keep labouring this point but it is impossible to overstress it. My belief is that what a woman in labour needs more than anything else is a sense of purpose in what she is doing, support, encouragement and the reminder that each contraction is playing its part in producing her baby. If she can keep this in her mind, with the idea of working *with* the muscle action of the uterus, her breathing pattern will automatically change with the needs of the moment.

OVERBREATHING

It must be emphasized how essential it is for the breathing to be kept as rhythmical and as physically effortless as possible. The effort is at the level of the will, the quiet determination to deal with just one contraction. There should never be any 'pumping' of the breath with exaggerated movements of the chest and shoulders. Blowing out and taking in breaths too strenuously for any length of time can result in an imbalance of carbon dioxide and oxygen in the bloodstream, and cause a condition known as hyperventilation.

The first sign of hyperventilation is a feeling of tingling in the fingers. If overbreathing is continued, the sense of numbness will extend up the arms and into the body and lead to a rigidity in the limbs and an inability to move. This can be very alarming for the person concerned. At any sign of hyperventilation, the most effective treatment is to hold a paper or plastic bag over the person's nose and mouth. Ask her to breathe rhythmically in and out. She will then be breathing back carbon dioxide, and the balance will usually quickly restore itself. Never hold the bag too tightly over the face. This could be alarming for the person concerned. And after every six or eight breaths take the bag away for a few moments. Provided a woman breathes easily and rhythmically, however, and allows her rate of breathing to change as the situation demands, no such problems should occur. Yet it is something a husband can watch for, and if his wife appears to be breathing with too much effort he can simply remind her to quieten it down.

COPING WITH PAIN

The end of the first stage is always the most difficult part of labour, and its importance should never be minimized. At this point pain is nearly always at its maximum and it can seem that there is no longer any pause between contractions. If the pain has been felt initially in the lower part of the abdomen, it often radiates to the back at this stage. Something that can help enormously to alleviate such pain in the back is for someone to apply firm pressure to the lower part of the spine.

A mere gentle rubbing is not much help, but as a contraction starts, pressing hard against the sacrum (the bones at the lower part of the spine where it joins the pelvic girdle) will sometimes relieve the pain quite astonishingly. Back pressure will usually

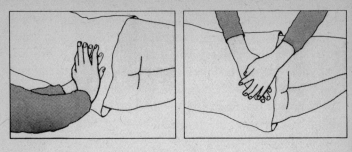

Fig. 7   Positions for helping hands.

help at any point during labour, and even where pain is felt only in the abdomen, pressure on the back can relieve it.

If the woman is lying on her side, the person doing the pressing can stand behind her and press hands firmly against her back. Or it can be very helpful to stand in front of her, lean over and pull on her back. An exceptionally firm pressure can be obtained in this way, with the added advantage that comes from facing her, and so maintaining an eye-to-eye contact and, if necessary, reminding her how to breathe. Some women cannot bear any pressure on their backs, but it is always worth trying, and in some cases can bring unbelievable relief. One girl, whom I taught for all her four pregnancies, insisted that she would never have been able to cope unless her husband had been there to press her back on each occasion. And he, somewhat ruefully, admitted that for several days after her deliveries his arms ached from unaccustomed strain on particular muscles.

Another important phenomenon of the end of the first stage of labour is the effect it can have on the emotions. This is the time when a woman can really lose her sense of humour! She may grow very weepy. Everything may seem to be getting on top of her. She may feel she cannot go on for much longer. She may also lose control of her language, and anyone sitting with a woman in labour should be warned of the possibility. A husband must be especially prepared, for he will undoubtedly be the one to receive the full force of her invective! As one girl wrote to me: 'Thank goodness you had warned them at the Fathers' Evening about the language we might use. Even so, my husband's jaw fell six feet. He didn't know I knew such words. I didn't either, but I found it very satisfying.'

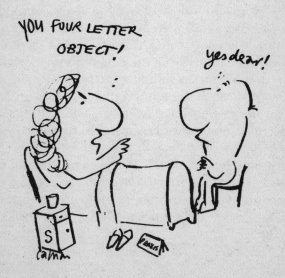

Women can feel very guilty over an unexpected emotional outburst at the end of the first stage, and men can be hurt and worried if they have not been forewarned of the possibility. But if they are prepared for it they will accept it cheerfully as a sign that the most difficult period of labour is nearing its conclusion.

So many women say what a blessed relief it is to be able to realize that the feeling of desperation and inability to carry on much longer indicates that the end is in sight. But it is hard for a woman in labour to be completely objective at this point, and so it can help if she is reminded that the end is near.

One woman who had had several children told me: 'That moment when I felt ready to give up was a shining signpost on my road of labour, telling me that I was almost there. It was always a tremendous boost to my morale when my husband reminded me that, because I was saying that I couldn't go on for much longer, it meant that I didn't have to.'

At this point in labour it is more important than ever that a woman should cope with the contractions *one by one*. If she starts trying to anticipate how many more there may be to go, she will lose her concentration on the one she is dealing with *here and now*.

For some women, the last part of this stage of labour is not prolonged, for others it lasts longer. There are so many factors, including the position of the baby, over which no one has any control.

THE URGE TO PUSH

In due course a woman will feel increasing pressure into the pelvis, until it becomes a bearing-down sensation and she will have a strong urge to push. This expulsive desire can be extremely embarrassing for a woman who has had no explanation beforehand, for it feels just the same as a compulsive bowel movement. Many women who have had no ante-natal preparation, and so do not understand the reason for it, tense up with shame against this uncontrollable urge to bear down, and by so doing only make their situation the more difficult.

The bearing-down sensation is, in fact, nature's way of making a woman assist in the birth of her baby by holding her breath and pushing with the expulsive uterine contractions. It is to be greeted with relief, for it is always a sign that the cervix is reaching full dilation. It is completely involuntary, and often shows itself by a woman holding her breath and grunting. *Any suggestion of her wanting to push must be reported at once to the midwife, if she is not present at the time. She should not start pushing until she has been told that she may do so.*

This is because it quite often happens that a woman begins to have a desire to push before the cervix is fully dilated. This is caused when the back part of the cervix pulls up more quickly than the front part, which allows the baby's head to press against the back passage, and sends a nervous stimulus that creates the expulsive urge before the front part of the cervix has stretched completely open. When this condition occurs (it is known as an 'anterior lip'), it can prove difficult and frustrating. The involuntary desire to bear down can be very strong, but the woman must not be allowed to give way to this urge until the lip of the cervix has disappeared.

The breathing that can carry her on, through this stage, if it happens, is our old friend huffing and puffing. This will prevent her holding her breath, and a woman has to be holding her breath before she can bear down. Some women find an inhalant pain reliever useful at this point in labour, and the use of this is described more fully in Chapter 9.

Thus the transition between the first and second stages ends with full dilatation of the cervix, when a woman having a hospital delivery will be taken to the delivery room, if she has not been transferred there earlier. She will now be allowed to push, and preparations will be put in hand for the actual birth of the baby.

Sometimes during the course of labour a woman can experience attacks of shivering. Her whole body may shake quite uncontrollably. These attacks, should they occur, usually do not last very long, but they can be unpleasant as well as alarming for both mother and father if they have not been forewarned of this possibility. There is little to be done. The more she tries to stop herself from shaking and shivering, the more she will be aware of it. She must try to relax as much as possible and wait for it to wear off. But it can be very comforting for her at such moments to have a hand to hold and a few words of re-assurance.

# 8

# The Second Stage of Labour

Once full dilatation has been achieved and a woman is allowed to push, the end of her labour is in sight. This second stage of labour can be very exciting. It seldom lasts longer than one hour, and although it may prove very hard work, most women find it highly satisfying. Now at last, a woman feels she can do something active to expedite the birth of her baby. Up to this point all that she has been able to do 'has been to stay relaxed, breathe through each contraction and wait patiently for the cervix to dilate. But from now on her own physical effort will play a very important part in the delivery of her child.

The first requirement of the second stage is for the woman to be in the correct position. It is essential that she be propped up on pillows and *not* left lying flat on her back. If she is completely flat, it will be impossible for her to push correctly since she will then find that her chin is tilted upwards and most of her energy wasted by straining into her throat. But if she is supported by pillows at an angle of approximately forty-five degrees, she will be able to round her shoulders and tuck her chin down on to her chest; and then she will be able to direct all her muscular effort towards bringing about the birth.

I always feel strongly that there should be no compulsion on a man either to be or not to be with his wife during delivery. This is a highly personal decision that should be left to those concerned: the husband and wife as well as the doctor and midwife. Sometimes obstetrical reasons may make it inconvenient or undesirable for the husband to remain, but so long as everything is progressing normally and a man wishes to be present when his child is born, there is every reason why he should be allowed to do so. A majority of doctors and midwives today will be quite willing for the husband to stay if he so wishes, always provided they can see that the man is being of help to his wife, and know that he will co-operate with them by doing as he is asked without question. Indeed, one absolute condition for the husband's presence with his wife during labour should be that, if he is asked to go, he will do so without hesitation.

The sharing of the actual moment of birth can be a profoundly moving experience for a husband and wife, and help to cement the foundation of their new three-way family relationship. But if the husband does not wish to be there, this too should be his freedom of choice, and no one should make him feel guilty, or that he has failed in any way. Where the husband *is* present, however, it is important for him to understand the role he can play and the way he can positively help his wife. For a start he can make sure she is supported comfortably on pillows, and ask for extra ones if necessary.

The contractions of the second stage are of an expulsive nature, and feel like a compulsive desire to evacuate the bowels. As a woman feels each one starting, she will pick up her legs, hold her thighs, take in a deep breath and hold it. Then, with her shoulders rounded and her chin tucked down, she must push with the contraction towards her rectum. The secret of pushing correctly, and so of gaining the maximum effect from each contraction, is to push *long* with a quiet will and a determination to push the baby down and out. Pushing a baby down can be very hard work, but it is important for the mother to think 'push long' rather than 'push hard'. It is the long, protracted pressure from above that is far more effective than short, hard pushes.

An innate fear in many women is apt to inhibit their effort at this point. They become afraid that if they push too much they will hurt themselves. Often a bulging, burning sensation is felt as the baby's head stretches the muscular outlet (the perineum), and women feel that they may split open. But there is no need for this fear. The obstetric team will be watching very carefully, and, if necessary, an incision will be made into the perineum to relieve the strain on the muscles of the pelvic floor. (This very minor operation is known as an 'episiotomy'.) A woman who holds herself back from pushing with her full will is only delaying the delivery. So she must continue to take in a deep breath, hold it, close her mouth, tuck her chin

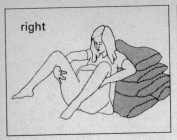

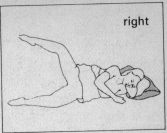

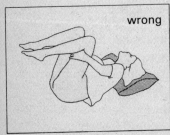

Fig. 8    Positions for the
second stage of labour.

down and *push* for as long as she can. If when she lets
her breath go the contraction is still present, she
must take in another breath and push again. She
should be able to do two or three pushes to a
contraction, depending on how long each one lasts.
It can be, as I say, very hard work. Your wife will
become very red in the face as she pushes, and as she
releases her breath she will grunt. If either she or
you are unprepared for this, it can come as an
embarrassing shock, but with both of you forewarned and knowing what to do, she can get on
with her job with a sense of achievement, while you
can encourage her in her work.

More often than not it takes two or three
contractions for the woman to get into the rhythm

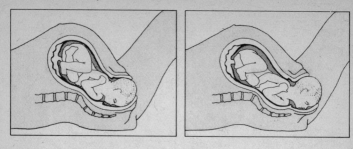

Fig. 9  Progress of the second stage.

of pushing. A few more contractions and the baby's head will begin to show at the height of the contraction. What an exciting moment it is when the doctor or midwife says: 'We can see your baby's head.' After all those months the baby is actually in sight! As one girl told me: 'I could hardly believe it. The bulge was becoming a person, and he had black hair.' (In actual fact it turned out to be a 'she' with long dark curls.)

The husband who is present during the second stage will be standing by his wife's head, supporting her and encouraging her, and he will not be able to see any of the physical details unless he wants to look. I stress this because men are so often afraid that they will inevitably become involved in the actual delivery, and imagine a situation that bears no relation to fact. At the birth a woman's legs and abdomen will be covered with sterile sheets, and these will screen the actual birth of the baby from the eyes of those at the head of the bed. On the other hand if either the mother or father wish to watch the baby emerging, they can do so, but the choice is theirs.

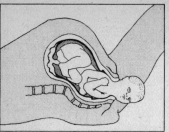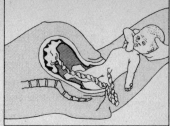

Fig. 10    Delivery completed.

A man can help considerably if, as a contraction starts, he puts an arm behind his wife's shoulders and lifts her forward. Being supported in this way, she can more easily keep her chin tucked down, and this will help her to push correctly. At the same time he can remind her to 'push *long... long...*'. One long push always achieves far more than ten short pushes. The midwife, who will be present right the way through the second stage, will help her to hold up her legs as she pushes; or, in hospital they may sometimes be supported in stirrups. At the end of each contraction your wife will lie back on her pillows and breathe deeply in and out, gathering herself for the effort of the next contraction. It can be very refreshing and comforting for her to have her face wiped with a cool, damp sponge between contractions.

## THE DELIVERY

At the beginning of the second stage the baby's head is flexed, chin down on to his chest, and delivery is achieved by the head being pushed through the pelvic outlet and then extending over the perineum. The back of the baby's head is the first part to be delivered; this then extends upwards to reveal the forehead, eyes, nose, mouth and chin. As soon as the head is delivered the shoulders rotate so that the baby's body is lying sideways in the pelvis, which means that the shoulders and the body can now be delivered with comparative ease.

As the baby's head is being 'crowned' and delivered the mother will probably be asked to stop pushing to allow the doctor or midwife to deliver the head gently and slowly. Her response will be to breathe in and out quickly and fairly shallowly. This panting type of breathing will prevent her from pushing. Once the head is delivered, the difficult part of the second stage is over. She may be asked to push slightly, or to pant for the delivery of the shoulders, and then the baby's body will slide out immediately afterwards.

HOW THE BABY MAY LOOK

What a memorable moment this is. But it can be entirely spoiled if it is not understood how, at birth, a baby's body can be a bluish-purple colour. As soon as the baby cries, his lungs will expand and he takes in oxygen as his individual, separated circulation takes over. He will then turn a normal colour very quickly, but sometimes it is several minutes before this happens, and until then he can look very blue and limp. It can be extremely frightening for the mother if she has not been warned, and for the father, if he is present.

Another thing that should be known is that during pregnancy a foetus is covered with a white cheesy substance called 'vernix', which is actually a natural protective covering. This begins to wash off as a baby comes to term, but most babies still have a few patches of vernix on their bodies when they are born. There will probably also be some streaks of blood on the head and body, but this does not indicate any damage to the baby. Having a baby is, in fact, a far less messy business than most people imagine, though there is bound to be a slight loss of blood, and traces will inevitably adhere to the baby's body as he is delivered.

Expectant parents should be warned too of the possible appearance of the genitals of the new born. During pregnancy the developing foetus absorbs hormones from the mother's body, and this often causes enlargement of the genitals at birth. The vulva of a baby girl is often swollen, but this is not as noticeable as the scrotum of a new-born boy, which can be enlarged and look very blue. This can prove very alarming for the mother and father if they have not been forewarned of this possibility. They settle down to a normal size and colour fairly quickly, but many new parents have expressed appreciation and relief of understanding the nature of this phenomenon.

IMMEDIATE ATTENTION TO THE BABY

As soon as the baby has been born the midwife may

aspirate the upper respiratory passages to make sure that no mucus is caught there to interfere with his respiration. This she does by passing a small tube down his throat and up his nose so that she can suck any mucus out. It is a NORMAL procedure and does not mean that anything is wrong. There is always oxygen and everything for resuscitation on hand if anything is required, but it is seldom needed. However, it is comforting to know that every modern obstetric and pediatric device is available if the baby should need any special attention. New-born babies usually start to cry spontaneously and the traditional slap on the behind to start them off is now a thing of the past. The midwife will also have checked the precise time of the baby's birth at this point so that it can be recorded. If things have been busy, the husband can help by remembering or jotting it down.

The next thing to be done is for the doctor or midwife to cut the umbilical cord. There are no nerves in the cord, so it is not painful for either mother or baby. Two or three clamps are attached to the cord, and with a pair of scissors it is simply cut between these clamps. The piece of umbilical cord that remains attached to the baby's navel is then left in position. It will usually shrivel and fall away by the time the baby is about a week old. The other end of the cord comes away with the placenta during the third stage of labour.

If a mother wishes to hold her baby as soon as he is born, she should have no hesitation in asking to do so, and if her husband is present he can make the request for her. Some mothers feel very nervous about holding a new-born baby, and no woman should be made to feel guilty if she does not want to touch her baby immediately. Sometimes the reluctance to handle a baby as soon as he is born springs from the idea that he is very fragile and might come to some harm. But if a baby is placed on his mother's abdomen or given to her to hold, she will soon realize how very strong he is.

THE AFTERBIRTH

The third stage of labour is the expulsion of the placenta, and is usually completed ten to fifteen minutes after the delivery of the baby. A woman will sometimes be asked to give a gentle push, but on the whole there is little more she can do. She has played her part and should feel satisfied with her efforts. It remains only to insert any stitches if these have been made necessary by an episiotomy. This takes approximately twenty to thirty minutes, depending on how many stitches are needed. Once this has been completed, the mother will be sponged, changed and, if in hospital, transferred from the delivery room back to her bed.

# 9

# Analgesics and Anaesthetics

## ANALGESICS

It will be useful, and may save you a few
misapprehensions, if you have some previous
knowledge of the kind of analgesic aid that will be
available for your wife during her labour should she
need it for any reason. Analgesics are simply pain-
relieving drugs. They may be administered by
injection, or as a gas through an inhalant
apparatus.

Once labour is well established in the first stage,
with the contractions regular and building up more
strongly, a woman may feel that she needs some
help to counteract the pain. She will then probably
be given an injection. Within ten to fifteen minutes
she will begin to feel drowsy, with a sense of well-
being and euphoria that most women find pleasant.
The injection will not have eliminated the pain
completely, and it would be unfair to suggest
otherwise. But it will have taken the edge off it, and
the degree of relaxation that it induces can
certainly be helpful. The initial effect will last for
three to four hours, and then, depending on the
pattern of labour and the stage reached, she will, if

necessary, be given another injection.

The only drawback is that some women find that the drug has a disorienting effect and interferes with their concentration and breathing during contractions. When a husband is present, his help may therefore be invaluable as he reminds his wife what she should do. He should make his wife open her eyes and look at him when a contraction starts, and if he does the breathing himself, she will then be able to follow it and so will be helped to maintain her concentration.

Where an inhalant analgesic is used, it will be self-administered and the woman will always be shown how to use the apparatus. As a contraction starts, she will hold the mask tightly over her nose and mouth and breathe in and out, deeply and regularly. When the contraction is over she should remove the mask and breathe quite normally. When using the mask is the *only* time that she should breathe deeply during a contraction, for deep breathing is essential to absorb an effective amount of the drug. Apart from this she should never, of course, breathe deeply down into her abdomen during a contraction, but always try to keep in her mind the idea of breathing 'above' the pain.

Some women find an inhalant analgesic a great help; others cannot tolerate it because they cannot stand anything covering their faces, and find that it interferes with their concentration on their breathing. When this happens, there is no reason for a woman to feel impelled to use the apparatus. There are no inflexible rules about what should or should not be done; about what may or may not help. All a woman can do is wait until the moment arrives and then accept the help that is available to her when or if she needs it. An inhalant analgesic is most likely to be used during the end of the first stage of labour, though it is sometimes also used during the second stage.

## EPIDURAL ANAESTHESIA

Epidural anaesthesia is an effective, well-tested method of achieving almost, if not completely, painless childbirth whilst remaining fully conscious. The technique depends on injecting local anaesthetic into the epidural space that surrounds the outer covering of the spinal cord to anaesthetize the nerves that carry pain stimuli to the brain. A very fine, hair-like plastic tube is inserted into the epidural space, and it is through this tube that the anaesthetic is introduced. The tube is strapped to the woman's back and left in position so that the anaesthetic can be 'topped up' when it wears off and pain recurs. The tube is so fine that a woman can lie on her back without being aware of it, though in practice she will often be asked to lie on her side to help stabilize her blood pressure since this can be lowered by the administration of epidural anaesthesia. To prevent this, it is usual when an epidural is administered, to set up an intravenous drip of a solution which helps to stabilize the blood pressure.

This can be alarming for both mother and father

if they have not been prepared for it, as indeed can be the use of monitoring machines. These machines are used to monitor the frequency, strength and duration of the contractions and also the rate of the baby's heart beat. Always be sure to have the working of the monitoring machine explained to you, so that you understand what it is signifying. Once you understand, you can watch it with interest and will be able to recognise any change that should be reported.

It is sometimes thought that a woman given an epidural anaesthetic will inevitably have a forceps delivery. This is not true. Many hundreds of woman have pushed their babies out by their own efforts when under epidural anaesthetic. It helps here if a woman has been taught the correct way of pushing, and then, in the second stage of labour, when a contraction starts and she is told to push, she will know exactly what to do.

Many women find they can move their legs quite easily with this type of anaesthetic, but some feel their legs grow heavy and numb. The latter sensation can be worrying for someone who has not been warned of the possibility. The effects of the anaesthetic usually wear off within a few hours of delivery and the woman will then be back to normal.

Occasionally it happens that the epidural does not work completely and affects only one side of the body. This can lead to a freakish lop-sided sensation: pain on one side and nothing on the other. Under such circumstances it can help a woman tremendously if she has her breathing techniques to fall back on.

Many women are under the impression that if they are going to have an epidural they will not need to learn anything about labour itself. They think that pain is the only aspect of labour that has to be contended with, and that so long as the pain is controlled by an epidural, that is all that will matter. This is a foolish and short-sighted assumption. A woman's understanding of the whole process of labour, of what is going on about her, of how to push correctly, and so on, will all help to reinforce her self-confidence and that sense of positive purpose that will be so important to her sense of well-being.

## GENERAL ANAESTHESIA

General anaesthetics are sometimes used in labour if a forceps delivery or a Caesarean Section become necessary. However, either of these may be done under epidural anaesthetic if possible. (See also page 101). If a woman should need a general anaesthetic, her husband will be asked to wait outside the delivery room. It can be very alarming for someone with no professional medical experience to see someone else being put under general anaesthesia, and as has already been emphasized, if it becomes necessary to ask a husband to leave, he must do so without hesitation or argument.

# THE BENEFITS OF ANALGESIA AND ANAESTHESIA

There is some controversy about the principle of administering analgesics and anaesthetics at all during labour. Some people still have the notion that if a woman does not suffer in some way during childbirth, if she does not 'go through it', she will fail to appreciate her child later on. This is utter, archaic nonsense. Others think that there is some special virtue in achieving a delivery without recourse to any drugs. This can be a very tense attitude. If a woman goes into labour determined to maintain a certain standard, it can easily cause tensions that may make the need for drugs even greater. Women should applaud the advance of medical science and accept with confidence and gratitude the help that modern analgesics and anaesthetics can offer them. The need for these will be kept to the minimum, and the minimum will have the maximum effect when given to the woman who is relaxed, confident and willing to accept whatever help she may need as her labour progresses.

There can be the fear among women of the effect that drugs and analgesics can have on the baby. It is quite true that the baby can be affected by analgesic drugs, but this fact is known to doctors and they watch very carefully to keep the amount within the safety limits.

# 10

# Delivery by Forceps, Vacuum Extraction or Caesarean Section

## FORCEPS AND THE VENTOUSE

Sometimes a situation arises that makes it necessary to deliver the baby by forceps, or by vacuum extraction. The position or size of the baby can, for instance, make it impossible for a woman to push her baby out by her own efforts. Should this happen, she must accept the help that obstetrical skill can give her with gratitude and without any sense of failure. Her desire to push her baby out by herself must always be balanced by common sense and the realization that this is not always possible. People think of forceps as 'damaging' and 'dangerous', but one must remember that they can be life-saving instruments. If she should need help with the birth of her baby, she should *never* feel that it is she who has failed, but rather that obstetrical skill has succeeded in the safe delivery of her child.

If forceps are needed they are always used under some form of anaesthetic, and sometimes the husband will be asked to leave the delivery room, especially if a general anaesthetic has to be administered.

The idea of a baby being delivered by vacuum extraction, the ventouse, can be very alarming if the simplicity of the procedure is not understood. It is simply a modern alternative to the use of forceps. A metal cup is attached to the baby's head inside the vagina by means of a vacuum created by a special apparatus, and when traction is applied it brings the baby's head down the birth canal. It is most important for both mother and father to know that, following a vacuum extraction, there will always be a swelling on the baby's head where the cup was applied. This swelling will disappear within a few hours, but a bruise may be left, which can remain for a while longer. Like the marks sometimes left by a forceps delivery, the bruise offers absolutely no cause for concern and will in due course disappear completely.

## CAESAREAN SECTION

Over the years a Caesarean Section has become a highly safe operation and will be performed where there is any indication that a vaginal delivery could put either mother or baby at risk.

Some circumstances will make a doctor decide to perform a Caesarean before a woman goes into labour. This is known as an elective Caesarean Section. There will also be the occasions when a situation arises during labour which will necessitate a Caesarean.

One indication for an elective Caesarean may be the position in which a baby is lying. If a baby is presenting breech, i.e. bottom down instead of head down, a Caesarean may be performed. There are means by which the measurements of a woman's pelvis can be accurately assessed. If these are adequate for the size of the baby the baby may be delivered buttocks and legs first. But if there were any doubt about this then the baby would be delivered by Caesarean Section.

Sometimes, where a baby is presenting breech, a doctor will turn the baby around. This is done externally with the woman lying on the examination couch and, using both hands, the doctor will rotate the baby until the head is down. Whether or not this version (as it is called) is performed will depend on the size of the pelvis, the size of the baby, the amount of water and the woman's obstetrical history. It must always be left to the doctor's discretion.

Occasionally a baby will lie transversely – across the mother's abdomen. There is only one course to follow in this situation – a Caesarean. Also if a woman has too small a pelvis for the baby's head to come through, or if it is deemed wise on account of her obstetrical history, then an elective Caesarean will be decided upon.

The commonest reasons for a Caesarean to be performed during labour are if the cervix does not open up completely or if the baby's heart shows signs of distress. Sometimes it happens that even with good, strong contractions a cervix does not dilate fully. Without full dilatation of the cervix it is impossible to deliver a baby vaginally. The only answer is a Caesarean.

The baby's heart is being monitored all through labour either with a foetal stethoscope or by a monitoring machine. The heart rate will often fluctuate during a contraction and cause no concern but any sign of continued 'foetal distress' will be noted and may be an indication for a Caesarean to be performed.

Today many Caesareans are done under epidural anaesthesia. This will depend on the wishes of the woman herself, the surgeon, the anaesthetist and the circumstances. The advantages of a Caesarean under epidural are that a mother is conscious at the moment of birth (although feeling nothing), and can hear her baby's first cry. Also, if a husband wishes to sit with his wife during the operation he is very often allowed to do so. If this circumstance arose and you wished to be with her, it is important to ask if you may do so. Otherwise, with all that is going on you might be forgotten! It must be added that neither mother nor father can see the Caesarean being performed. The sterile sheets which are placed over the woman's abdomen and the screen which is positioned over the upper part of the chest will block off any sight of the actual operation.

Should a woman undergo Caesarean section it is as well for her to be forewarned of the great discomfort she will feel for the first few days after the operation. But even this can be greatly mitigated if she resists the temptation to lie still in bed and feel sorry for herself. She must move her legs about in bed, and as soon as she gets up (which she will be made to do within twenty-four hours of the operation), she must try to stand as straight as possible and then to make herself walk as normally as she is able. It will not be easy, but it will pay many dividends, for moving about stimulates the circulation, prevents post-operative stiffness and reduces to a minimum post-operative wind pains. A few words of reminder and encouragement from her husband can help her tremendously in her resolve.

## THE SPECIAL CARE UNIT

If the baby has been under any stress during delivery, it is not uncommon to put the baby in the special care unit where he or she will be watched carefully. This can be very alarming for parents if they do not understand the procedures of modern pediatrics. It does not imply that there is anything wrong with the baby. But taking the precaution of keeping a baby under observation for a few hours helps to ensure the baby's well-being.

Mothers can be very worried that if they do not have immediate contact with their babies it will affect adversely a future relationship between the mother and her child. Of course it is good if a mother can fondle her baby as soon as possible, and it is not right that a baby should be separated from his mother immediately after birth for no good reason. But balance is a very important factor in life, and situations must be kept in proper perspective. If, for the sake of the baby's health and well-being, he needs to be in the special care unit it will not cause a problem in relationships. I have known a number of instances where premature babies have needed to be in an incubator for several weeks, and as they have grown up have still enjoyed a very close, secure relationship with both mother and father.

# PART III

# The Post-natal Period

# 11

# The After-effects of Childbirth

And so the baby is born. The build-up to labour, the natural anxieties that everyone experiences, the strain and hard work of labour itself – all this is over. It is an emotional moment to which every new mother reacts in a different way. Some are elated; some burst into tears and cry uncontrollably without knowing why; for others it comes as an anticlimax, and they feel a sense of lethargy and disinterest. Each woman must accept whatever *her* reactions are as normal.

There are many women who have no sense of reality about the baby and no feeling of overwhelming 'mother love' for several weeks after the birth. They may then feel guilty about their lack of maternal warmth towards the infant, feeling it to be wrong and unnatural and an indication that they will not make good mothers. None of this is true. The aftermath of birth brings with it a whole gamut of emotions, and no woman knows how she will react until the situation arises. Men, too, can be affected in different ways, and they should not be surprised if their pleasure, pride and great relief is countered by the deep fatigue and sense of anticlimax that so often follows a demanding emotional experience.

There now follow three very important months. It is true that the birth of the baby brings to an end the nine months of pregnancy but, at the same time, it ushers in a new period of adjustment for which both man and woman should be prepared. The three months following a baby's birth, particularly the first month, besides being joyous and exciting, can also be a difficult and testing time. The baby has brought a fresh dimension into the life of the new mother and father. Additional and unfamiliar responsibilities become a part of life, and certain freedoms have to be sacrificed. Sometimes they wonder if life can ever be the same again.

The answer to that is that life never will be the same again. It has changed, and it is not always easy to adapt to great changes. For the husband, the pleasures and difficulties of the post-natal period may be brought into proper perspective if he is prepared for the upheaval that the baby's arrival can cause, and for the effects that the birth can have on his wife, physically, emotionally and mentally.

## FATIGUE

No woman believes, until she experiences it, the intensity that post-natal fatigue ran reach. This is no general tiredness to be remedied by a few early nights and a little rest. It involves a total depletion of energy, and many women feel guilty because they are not able to resume a normal life on their return home from hospital. They think they should

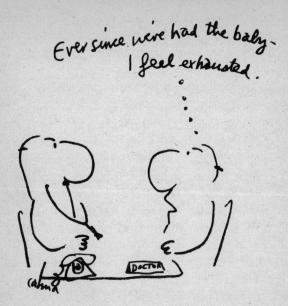

be able to integrate the new baby into the running of the home just like that, while preparing meals, shopping, entertaining and so forth, as though no cataclysmic change had occurred. But it will take time for her hormone balance to be re-established, and for her to adjust emotionally and mentally to being a mother. So many problems of the post-natal period would be reduced beyond measure if only those concerned could recognize this from the start. Wise are those who treat the first three months as a time of learning and adapting to a new situation.

The prime need to bring about this adjustment is, so far as the mother is concerned, rest. For the first six weeks, and preferably for the first two months, she should rest each day, if possible for at least one hour. Many women think that sitting down and 'putting their feet up' for half an hour constitutes a rest. They feel guilty about actually going to bed and lying down and sleeping when jobs are waiting to be done. But the new mother must get her priorities right. Washing, ironing, dusting, cooking, polishing are *not* as important as her health. Sitting in a chair with her feet up will *not* give her the same rest as lying down and relaxing completely. If she tries to do too much too soon, she will only prolong the period of her fatigue.

Even those women normally blessed with an abundance of energy are not immune to the effects of post-natal fatigue. A man's help to his wife during this period can be incalculable if he understands the situation and encourages her to rest and to leave undone the less important tasks. In the final analysis, everyone will be much happier if they can accept a certain amount of disruption to the normal smooth running of the home. Meals will often be a bit late; polished surfaces will not shine as they did before pregnancy; washing, ironing, mending will not be completed with the regularity that existed before the baby arrived.

But none of this will matter so long as it is accepted with a modicum of humour and humility by the woman who finds it impossible to get everything accomplished; and by the man who has to suffer the inconveniences.

Many women have a martyr-like compulsive

sense of perfection. Such a woman will drop with fatigue rather than leave one small task undone, but in trying to achieve her goal she only makes problems for herself and everyone round her. The more she tries to do, the more tired she becomes; the more tired she is, the greater the burden of the next job; and so she goes into a new sort of vicious circle. Every small hitch assumes gigantic proportions; she imagines she must be failing in her duty and pushes herself even harder. Her tension and fatigue react on everyone round her, and possibly even on the baby itself during the important early days when a basic sense of security is being established. If she continues in this vein, disaster will follow.

Every human being must accept some degree of limitation, and never is this more important for a woman than in those first months after she has had a baby. She *must* keep a proper sense of values, and be willing to leave undone the inessential jobs. If she tries to force herself to do too much before her full energy is restored, she will build problems for herself, her husband and her baby.

People do not always realize to what extent even small babies can be affected by the emotions of the people who handle them. A mother who is tense, tired and anxious will evoke a response in her baby, and he will probably be fretful. Equally, the more relaxed and unfatigued she is, the less nervous she will be, and the more of a soothing effect she will have on him. It is inevitable that a new mother will be tired, and she will be bound to feel anxious until she has become confident in her ability to care for her baby. But the problem can be kept to a minimum and an equilibrium maintained so long as she *rests* and thus prevents a normal fatigue from escalating to a point of exhaustion.

## VISITORS

Visitors can be a very mixed blessing, whether the baby has been delivered at home or in hospital.

There is always a good deal of excitement after a baby has been born. Flowers, telegrams and presents arrive. Adoring grandparents, relatives and friends, flock to pay their respects and admire the new arrival. Few people realize how exhausting conversation can be, especially when it is inevitably the same conversation over and over again. Everyone who comes expresses the same sentiments, and the mother replies in the same way. By the end of the day her already depleted energy will have been drained even more dramatically. Her visitors go home feeling cheerful and on top of the world and leave her in a state of sometimes near collapse.

This is no exaggeration, and any doctor or midwife will testify to many such examples. If the new mother is in hospital, the routine there does not allow for much rest anyway, and it is most important for her to take every opportunity to relax and rest and replace some of her lost energy before the time comes for her to leave. I am not suggesting that she should have no visitors. Of course she will want to see her family and friends, but they should be limited and should never stay too long.

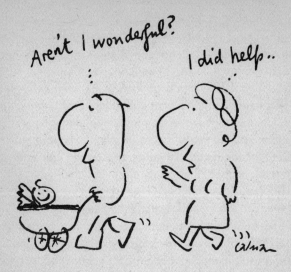

A husband can help with this. If he sees that his wife is tired from too many visitors, at home or in hospital, it is easier for him than for her to veto visits tactfully, or ask visitors not to stay too long. At home during the early days, visitors should continue to be restricted, especially those who have to be entertained. I need say no more on this subject except to quote from a letter that I received from one new mother:

The baby is a full-time job. Friends and family who offer to help should be taken at their word and given tasks to do and the new mother mustn't feel guilty at having lots of rest and generally ignoring any household problems that emerge. Husbands can help by gently dissuading people who want to visit from coming in the first two or three days or staying too long. It's the last time a new mother wants to entertain and the best friends are those who come for an hour, do the ironing or cook the dinner, then go!

## POST-NATAL DEPRESSION

Few women escape bouts of post-natal depression –
the 'maternity blues', as they are often called.
Often it is on the third or fourth day after delivery
that the new mother will suddenly feel weepy and
spend the day crying. It can prove very upsetting
for a husband who has not been warned of the
probability, especially since it is often his appearance that triggers off the tears.

She wonders why she had the baby; she knows
she will not be a good mother; she feels enveloped in
a black cloud, and it is difficult for her to glimpse
even the possibility of a silver lining. The worst
thing that anyone can do at this point is to try to
force her out of her mood, to try to 'make her see
reason', 'snap out of it', and 'pull herself together',
or even to start being jolly in an exaggerated sort of
way. All this will only exacerbate the situation.

The 'maternity blues' are a normal reaction to
birth – the release of several months of apprehension – and the new mother must be allowed to cry.
Tears are a great release of tension, and everyone
would be happier if only they realized that this was
so. But both men and women in our society are
indoctrinated during childhood with the idea that
crying is a sign of weakness, and so they deprive
themselves of an emotional safety valve that nature
has provided for them. The proverbial 'stiff upper
lip' only intensifies the emotional strain, sometimes
to a point of breakdown. Childbirth apart, it is high
time that people recognized the therapeutic effect

of tears. A new mother should be encouraged to cry, and reassured of the normality of such a reaction.

Once a mother is at home, the days of depression will come and go. It sometimes happens that new mothers, especially if before pregnancy they were leading busy lives and pursuing a career, will feel lonely and isolated at this time. Most women will, from time to time, feel resentment towards the baby, who has arrived to dominate their lives and restrict their freedom. How comforting it is for them to know that this is a normal reaction and nothing about which to feel guilty. It takes time to adjust to a new rôle, and entering the rôle of mother is the biggest change that a woman can experience in her life. The probationary period is bound to present difficulties alongside the rewards.

The days of being depressed will fluctuate over the first few weeks as the hormonal balance is adjusted, and after that the depression disappears. Over-fatigue will always exacerbate depression, which is another reason why rest is so absolutely essential. But if a woman finds she is having bouts of depression that are prolonged, if she is waking up early and cannot get back to sleep, or is generally being adversely affected by it, she should get in touch with her doctor. Women are so often reluctant to ask for help in these circumstances. They look on it as failure if they cannot rise above their depression. It is very foolish, however, for a new mother to try to fight on her own a situation that can today so often be relieved by simple medication. The longer she tries to fight depression by herself, the more tired she will become, and this in turn will intensify the depression.

Not all babies sleep right through the night during the first few months, and usually a mother will have to get up to attend to her child whenever he wakes. Broken sleep will aggravate fatigue, and sometimes a mild sedative is all that is needed to restore equilibrium. There is no shame in asking for the help that medical science can give. A husband will soon be aware if these problems do arise, and if his wife refuses to get in touch with her doctor, he should do so himself. *This is important.* There are occasions when a woman's reluctance to ask for medical aid should be overruled by positive action on her husband's part. By taking the initiative and seeking advice, he will be helping the family as a whole.

## SEX AFTER CHILDBIRTH

There is no medical reason why sexual relations should not begin again as soon as the couple desire, but, for a majority, it will benefit their sex lives if full sexual intercourse is delayed until the perineum has healed completely from the effects of stitches (see episiotomy page 84). Although this often takes several weeks medical advice should be sought if the problem persists over two months. If penetration by the penis is attempted too soon, the resulting pain can create great tension in the woman. Then, the next time intercourse takes place, she will recoil from the fear of pain, which will inevitably prevent her full participation and give neither partner satisfaction.

Fear of becoming pregnant again too soon is another factor in a woman's disinclination for sex, and it is imperative that she should seek professional advice on contraception as early as possible. It is very important to remember that breast feeding does not constitute a contraceptive. It is not probable that a woman will conceive while breast feeding, but it is perfectly possible.

Frigidity following a confinement is not uncommon, and it can last for several weeks, or even months. Such a loss of libido is often a result of postnatal fatigue or painful initial intercourse. Lovemaking must be very gentle when intercourse is resumed, and it is advisable to lubricate the vagina since the natural lubrication often does not return for some time and dryness in the vaginal lining makes penetration difficult and painful. Any spermicidal jelly or cream may be used. Great patience and tenderness is needed on both sides where any sexual problems do arise. It is as hard for the man as for the woman, perhaps even harder, but with love and patience any difficulties can usually be overcome in a few weeks. As a result, a deeper mutual understanding of one another's needs is often gained as a bonus. Sexual happiness between man and woman is an integral and important factor in their relationship.

If painful intercourse or loss of libido does persist, a woman should seek medical help, and the problem can usually be remedied without much difficulty. There are doctors who are trained in the specific work of counselling where sexual problems arise, and no one should hesitate to ask for help if it becomes necessary.

Sometimes a woman's lack of interest in sex can be caused by a combination of fatigue and preoccupation with the baby. The latter is understandable, but it is not always easy for her husband to accept. Most new mothers feel inadequate and anxious over their babies. They feel clumsy in handling the baby, and concerned that everything takes so long and that every waking hour is spent attending to the infant's needs and demands. Time and practice alone can give confidence to the new mother, and the reassurance that her husband understands her anxieties can relieve the feelings of guilt arising from any sense of divided loyalties. A mother who is breast feeding may feel she is spending too much time with the baby at the expense of her husband, but for her to give up breast feeding against her will and instincts can be more damaging to the relationship than adjustments that will usually be resolved within a few weeks.

A further word here is necessary about breast feeding. Some women do not want to breast feed and for others difficulties arise which make it impossible. The former should never be made to feel guilty. The latter will need comfort and understanding. A woman who wants to breast feed and cannot do so can feel very depressed and a failure. The calm support of the father will make all the difference to her acceptance of the situation.

A mutual recognition of feelings is essential, and open and frank discussions of them will help to keep the situation free from misunderstandings. Compromise is essential in every relationship throughout life, but it is never more important than between a husband and wife in the few months following the birth of a baby.

## THE NEW FAMILY UNIT

It is very important for a woman to remember that she is a wife as well as a mother. The husband – wife relationship is basic to family unity and something that must be nurtured. Because a baby has been born, it does not mean that romance is dead. In their new rôles of father and mother, the man and woman still remain lovers. The initial overwhelming emotion of being 'in love' may change as one grows older and situations in life alter, but changing situations can lead to greater maturity and deeper satisfaction.

As soon as the first few difficult weeks are over, and the new routine has been established, it is vital for the father and mother to have times alone together as husband and wife. It is a good idea for them to arrange for a reliable baby-sitter, in whom they have complete confidence, to come in for a few hours and allow them to go out by themselves away from the baby. For the mother it is a wonderful boost to her morale to be able to put on a pretty dress and get out to enjoy herself as a woman and a wife; and, for the father, it is pleasant to have his wife to himself for a little while.

Parents love their children, but they will love them that much more if they are able to get away from them for a short space of time every now and again. This benefits the children as much as parents. With the arrival of each new baby, the family unit grows and relationships within it change. Every new child has to be integrated into the family to become a part of the whole while yet maintaining his individuality and freedom. It is a great responsibility to have children, and a great challenge to take on the task of bringing them up. They must be guided through their early years and helped to develop through adolescence into a confident adulthood, when they will grow out of the family unit to live their own lives and, in due course, become parents themselves.

Parenthood starts with conception, and the mutual understanding and sharing of pregnancy. Childbirth and the months following it will help to build the firm foundation necessary for a family unit founded on love and emotional security. It is these two conditions above all that are so essential for the happiness of those who are involved in the positive and always developing situation that is family life.

# Index

# OTHER GREAT PAPERFRONT BOOKS

*Each uniform with this book*

## CROSSWORDS FOR THE ADDICT
## CROSSWORDS FOR THE DISCERNING

Alec Robins has been composing crosswords professionally for over 30 years. He appears in print in various guises: as 'Everyman' in *The Observer*, as 'Custos' in *The Guardian* and as 'Zander' in *The Listener*. A master of the art of the cryptic clue, he has assembled in these two books collections of his popular puzzles, mostly of the plain, 'armchair' type. And for those who like an occasional change a clutch of novelty is also included.

## CROSSWORDS FOR THE DEVOTEE
## CROSSWORDS FOR THE ENTHUSIAST

In these two books Don Putnam racks your brain with his concoctions of intelligence-strainers. Every cruciverbalist will find delight and entertainment from these puzzles, based on old familiars such as anagrams, charades, acrostics, riddles, spoonerisms etc. Why not slope your pen, don your thinking-cap, and accept the challenge?

# OUR PUBLISHING POLICY

## HOW WE CHOOSE

Our policy is to consider every deserving manuscript and we can give special editorial help where an author is an authority on his subject but an inexperienced writer. We are rigorously selective in the choice of books we publish. We set the highest standards of editorial quality and accuracy. This means that a *Paperfront* is easy to understand and delightful to read. Where illustrations are necessary to convey points of detail, these are drawn up by a subject specialist artist from our panel.

## HOW WE KEEP PRICES LOW

We aim for the big seller. This enables us to order enormous print runs and achieve the lowest price for you. Unfortunately, this means that you will not find in the *Paperfront* list any titles on obscure subjects of minority interest only. These could not be printed in large enough quantities to be sold for the low price at which we offer this series. We sell almost all our *Paperfronts* at the same unit price. This saves a lot of fiddling about in our clerical departments and helps us to give you world-beating value. Under this system, the longer titles are offered at a price which we believe to be unmatched by any publisher in the world.

## OUR DISTRIBUTION SYSTEM

Because of the competitive price, and the rapid turnover, *Paperfronts* are possibly the most profitable line a bookseller can handle. They are stocked by the best bookshops all over the world. It may be that your bookseller has run out of stock of a particular title. If so, he can order more from us at any time—we have a fine reputation for "same day" despatch, and we supply any order, however small (even a single copy), to any bookseller who has an account with us. We prefer you to buy from your bookseller, as this reminds him of the strong underlying public demand for *Paperfronts*. Members of the public who live in remote places, or who are housebound, or whose local bookseller is unco-operative, can order direct from us by post.

## FREE

If you would like an up-to-date list of all paperfront titles currently available, send a stamped self-addressed envelope to
ELLIOT RIGHT WAY BOOKS, BRIGHTON RD.,
LOWER KINGSWOOD, SURREY, U.K.